Is Your Sickness Real?

Is Your Sickness Real?
MIND-MADE DISEASE

The Helen Vale Foundation

Edited by
Shri Vijayadev Yogendra

MACMILLAN PUBLISHING CO., INC.
New York

Macmillan Publishing Co., Inc.
866 Third Avenue, New York, N.Y. 10022
Collier Macmillan Canada, Ltd.

Library of Congress Cataloging in Publication Data
Helen Vale Foundation.
Is your sickness real?
1. Medicine, Psychosomatic. I. Title.
RC49.H43 1978 616.08 78-18216
ISBN 0-02-621400-8

First American Edition 1978

Printed in the United States of America

Preface

WE ARE BECOMING increasingly aware that a great deal of ill-health in our community is related to our inability to live at peace with ourselves. We recognize disorders which we label psychosomatic because we see a direct link between this lack of inner harmony and disorded body function. In addition we are familiar with a host of diseases that result from disordered living, such as results from alcoholism, cigarette smoking, analgesic abuse and over-eating. We can extend it further into the medical consequences of socio-pathic behaviour manifested by battered babies and many road accidents.

We attempt to match this onslaught with a medical heritage based on simple notions of disordered organ function, specific causative agents and on treatment with the 'silver bullet' of Ehrlich.

Uneasily, we conclude that to deal with the medical problems of today we need a health-centred philosophy rather than the traditional disease-orientated teaching. Then we find that our own heritage is almost totally lacking in the raw material from which we can build that philosophy.

Little wonder we turn, however reluctantly, to examine how others have approached the problem. The critical point is concerned with the manner in which we attempt this task. Chairman Mao offered his colleagues the opinion that they should study the achievements of foreign peoples, and then adapt to Chinese needs that which they saw to be good. He emphasized two processes — selection and adaption — and saw clearly that to transplant anything in its entirety into another cultural framework would probably doom it to failure.

The authors contributing to this book have sought to integrate the familiar with the unfamiliar. The unfamiliar is exemplified by teachings long practised in Asia and long neglected by the West. The Western reader should judge how well the selection and adaptation process has been achieved by asking himself whether what he reads makes sense to him in familiar terms, which after all is the test he will apply without thinking to those authors who discuss problems in traditional Western format. The extent to which the East loses its mystery and mysticism is to me the measure of its impact.

Professor K. McLean
Associate Professor,
Monash University Department of Medicine,
Prince Henry's Hospital, Melbourne.
August 1977.

Foreword

I AM HAPPY TO NOTE that the Yoga Education Centre and The Helen Vale Foundation have published this work 'Mind-Made Disease'. The participation of eminent authors in this symposium will no doubt contribute greatly to the understanding of Eastern and Western viewpoints on the treatment of psychosomatic disorders. This blending and exchange of ideas will be most helpful to those, who are seeking, from both the East and West, ideas that will enable them to further their study of psychosomatic medicine.

Human problems are countless, and most of them are so interrelated personally and socially that no satisfactory or permanent solution can be found through any one or more sciences. It should also be realized that when man who cannot understand himself tries to understand another, he is surely going to make mistakes. Therefore, in trying to understand man the specialized sciences have been found wanting.

The old Western concept of body-mind parallelism has given way to what is now termed 'psychosomatics'. Unfortunately, while modern sciences are feverishly exploiting this new concept with curiosity, psychosomatics still suffers many disqualifications.

In India, Yoga as a science, both pure and exact, was

referred to as the ultimate remedy for all ailments of existential life. It thus accepted man as a whole and not as parts. In fact, Yoga is a total therapy of personality — physical, mental, moral, intellectual and spiritual — which operates and treats the total man and not his parts. Yoga therapy is a way of life, more general and less specific. Psychosomatics is a poor imitation of the universal Yoga concept of total therapy of personality.

Shri Yogendra
President,
International Board of Yoga.

Contents

PREFACE vii

FOREWORD ix

INTRODUCTION 1

PART ONE

Psychosomatics in Perspective

Background

Anxiety in Every Age 11
Professor David Maddison

Tension: The Basis of Psychosomatic Disease 20
Dr Alec Dempster

Emotional Education 26
Dr Satya Pal Duggal

On Psychosomatic Disease 31
Dr John Pawsey

Aspects of Treatment

Routines: The Basis of Health 37
Dr Jayadev Yogendra

Psychosomatic Techniques of Yoga 44
Dr David Mander/Patrick Dugan

On Psychosomatic Health Care 51
Jan Dugan

Psychosomatic Aspects of Dental Care 59
Dr Ronald French

Psychosomatics in Practice 66
Dr John Walters

The Practitioner

Character in Health 77
Janet Gudkovs

Humanity in Medicine 82
Kenneth Ingbritsen

Reflections of a Bystander 91
Dr John Funder

PART TWO
Psychosomatic Medicine: Eastern and Western Approaches

Is Yoga Healing or Therapy? 101
Shri Yogendra

Psychosomatic Disease in Ayurveda 106
Pandit Shiv Sharma

Psychosomatic Aspects of Traditional Chinese Medicine 114
Dr Yasuo Otsuka

Yoga Psychology 121
Dr C.T. Kenghe

Yoga Versus Psychology 137
Dr Robert Sherman

New Trends in Psychosomatic Medicine 147
Dr William Kroger

Psychosomatic Medicine 152
Dr Frank Graham

Morality and Psychosomatics 158
Shri Vijayadev Yogendra

BIOGRAPHICAL NOTES 175

GLOSSARY 181

INDEX 183

Introduction

WITH THE INCREASING interest in psychosomatic medicine and new developments in the fields of psychology and psychiatry, the Yoga Education Centre, Melbourne, and The Helen Vale Foundation felt they could make a contribution in the field of psychosomatics by bringing together papers and essays on the subject from both Eastern and Western viewpoints. The contributors discuss psychosomatic problems and offer some solutions as well. The book is not aimed at the academic-minded but at laymen who are interested in understanding diseases caused by psychological and emotional disturbance. The contributors come from both Eastern and Western traditions, their personal involvements are varied and wide and their experiences mature and reliable.

Today many people are trying to study the interrelationship between the psychological and physiological aspects of normal and abnormal body functions, and an attempt is being made to devise a form of therapy or psychotherapy that will enable an individual to overcome stress and cure conditions of psychosomatic disease. Though in the West the formal development of psychosomatic medicine began only in the early 1920's, the basic principles of psychosomatic medicine were available a few thousand years ago in the study of Ayurvedic medicine, Yoga technology and other Eastern life sciences.

The biggest challenge man faces today in problems of health is not overcoming contagious diseases, because they are well-contained and most of the world is free from them. However, the factor that is causing untold suffering throughout the world is psychosomatic disease, which has a lingering quality and is hard to overcome. These chronic, functional disorders take a very heavy toll on man.

The psychosomatic aetiology of disease is now being studied throughout the world by the behavioural scientists, psychologists and psychoanalysts, who are trying to find methods of modifying and controlling the emotions and so enhance the individual's control over his bodily functions. However, though man is a biological organism, the basic thesis for the study of man is not simple. It is no longer sufficient for medical science to understand the superficialities of health and biological control. It should also consider whether spiritual factors can cause or precipitate a disorder or disease. In the recently published book **Psychosomatic Medicine** by Doctors Lipowski, Lipsitt and Whybrow, it is stated: 'Psychosomatic medicine has had a four-fold meaning all along; as a science, as an approach to the prevention and treatment of physical illness, as a point of view on the nature of man and as a reformist movement in medicine.'(1) They go further to define psychosomatic medicine as firstly, a scientific study of the relationship between the psychological, social and biological factors in determining health and disease; secondly, as a holistic approach to the practice of medicine; and thirdly as consultation-liaison psychiatry. However, modern psychology, medicine and psychiatry have yet to accept that man is not only a physical entity but that he also has a soul, a psychic faculty, that overrides the mind-body complex. The Eastern authorities recognize this factor and see it as the source of psychosomatic disorders. Therefore, they accept ethical and moral values or spirituality as fundamental in overcoming conditions of a psychosomatic nature.

We believe that every medical practitioner — whether a specialist, a general practitioner or a psychiatrist — every psychologist, every counsellor and lay individual if given an opportunity to alleviate human suffering should be able to understand it at a deeper level through love and through his own spirituality. In so doing he can find solutions for his fellow human being who is suffering a profound deprivation and rejection of himself in this crisis-filled world.

In 1977 we were informed of the Fourth International Congress of Psychosomatic Medicine to be held in Kyoto, Japan. We were invited to participate and submit a paper for the proceedings. We were also informed that a special symposium on Yoga and psychosomatics was being held. At the same time The Helen Vale Foundation considered producing a special edition of the 'Journal of The Helen Vale Foundation' devoted entirely to the themes and needs of the Psychosomatic Congress. However, as the contributions started coming in, the idea grew and we found ourselves with much rich material on psychosomatic medicine. It was decided therefore not to bring out a special edition of the Journal but instead to produce a book containing all relevant articles as a reference work for people throughout the world. This volume is the result of that decision.

In the volume both Eastern and Western scholars and medical practitioners have explained their own approach to psychosomatic medicine by means of case histories, and their own tested theories on how psychosomatic progress can be achieved. This symposium gives us strength in believing that a total concept of psychosomatic medicine can be developed by allowing both Eastern and Western thinkers to find a new approach to the definition and treatment of psychosomatic problems.

The book is divided into two parts. Part One: 'Psychosomatics in Perspective' presents a general outline of psychosomatic health in three sections. The first section, 'Background', examines issues related to the development of psychosomatic problems. Topics include: 'Anxiety in Every Age', 'Tension: The Basis of Psychosomatic Disease', 'Emotional Education', and 'On Psychosomatic Disease'. The second section deals with aspects of treatment: 'Routines: The Basis for Health', 'Psychosomatic Techniques of Yoga', 'On Psychosomatic Health Care', 'Psychosomatic Aspects of Dental Care' and 'Psychosomatics in Practice'. The third section looks at the practitioner's role: 'Character in Health', 'Humanity in Medicine' and 'Reflections of a Bystander'. Part Two: 'Psychosomatic Medicine: Eastern and Western Approaches', brings together articles from eminent Eastern and Western authorities discussing trends and traditional approaches in psychosomatic medicine. Topics in this part include: 'Is Yoga Healing or Therapy?', Yoga Versus Psychology', 'Yoga Psychology', 'Psychosomatic Disease in Ayurveda', 'Psychosomatic Aspects of Traditional Chinese Medicine', 'New Trends in Psychosomatic Medicine', 'Psychosomatic Medicine' and 'Morality and Psychosomatics'.

It is hoped the book will be of practical value to both laymen and professionals. It has been prepared by people genuinely interested in finding answers, not for the sake of tying up solutions, but because more light on this subject is dearly needed. The volume, like the overall effort of the Foundation, aims to make a positive imprint on the lives of the people it touches.

The Helen Vale Foundation and The Yoga Education Centre wish to take the liberty of thanking each contributor for whose thoughts and knowledge we are deeply indebted. We would also like to thank Mr Paul Sumner, Mrs Sue Ellingsen, Mr Paul Howson, Mr Michael Findlay and others who have helped in the production of this book. We are happy to present this volume to the public as our contribution to the understanding of psychosomatic problems.

Shri Vijayadev Yogendra
Chairman,
The Helen Vale Foundation

1. Lipowski, Lipsitt & Whybrow, **Psychosomatic Medicine**, Oxford University Press, New York (1977)

Part One

Psychosomatics in Perspective

Background

Anxiety in Every Age

Professor David Maddison

JULES MASSERMAN once said: 'In the beginning was the word and the word was anxiety' — and if we can be certain of one thing, we can be certain that human beings will always be anxious, about this issue or that, for the basic roots of anxiety lie deep within our infantile and childhood experience, and no mere social revolution is going to abolish them. Pickling oneself in alcohol or pot, while waiting Micawber-like for something to happen, clearly does nothing to postpone the evil day. Changing the sexual rules, so that one reduces sex to sexology and tries to convert love to a lifelong masturbation fantasy based on an unrestricted diet of permissive magazines and TV shows may modify some sexual problems, while it induces or magnifies others — sexual anxiety was not made to be conquered by those with a simplistic turn of mind. As Andre Gide has said: 'To know how to free oneself is nothing — the arduous thing is to know what to do with one's freedom.'

The immense mass of information that we have at our disposal about the complexity of modern culture could be arranged under an almost infinite number of possible headings. I have chosen but two, 'Choice' and 'Detribalization'. I suspect that the exponentially increasing range of choices available to modern man, plus increasing pressure to participate in the business of choosing, lie at the root of a great deal of contemporary angst (fear), and will do so to an even greater extent in the future — at least until society regains its senses.

I always recognize that I am really back in North America, where the desirability of human choice has assumed a quite religious significance, when I buy my first snack lunch at the nearest delicatessen. Having decided which of the sixty-odd fillings will grace one's sandwich (and this would be about the end of it in Australia), many of you will recall that one is then, under immense pressure from both staff and fellow customers, forced rapidly into a positive orgy of inescapable decision-making: what type of bread? with butter or without? crusts on or off? what type of pickle within the sandwich? if mustard — what sort? what type of savory pickle on the plate? french fries or not? coffee 'regular' i.e. with cream — if so, what grade of cream? sugar? do you want it 'to go' — i.e., take away? By the time I stagger back on to the sidewalk I have lost my appetite, exhausted by this sudden exposure to a range of choices, nearly all of them attractive, reducing to helpless terror the untrained participant who began his mission with no intention other than that of buying what used to be called a ham sandwich.

And yet this vignette, I suggest, is not really too unrepresentative of many of the problems of modern living. Lipowski, in a series of provocative papers over the past four or five years, has likened the dilemma of modern man to that of Buridan's ass, who starved to death between two stacks of hay, unable to decide which of them to approach. Clearly man has always been faced with choices, and all concepts of healthy ego function would include, variously worded, some reference to the individual's ability to make reality-based decisions when faced with competing alternative pathways. But only since the eruption of aggressive advertising in the past few decades has man been bombarded almost continuously with information as to the range of options available to him, a problem which of course has only been compounded in this country by the monstrous, wildly disproportionate growth of commercial television, which ensures that nobody is immune — and there is evidence to suggest, patterns of television viewing being as they are, that the less one is capable of coping effectively, the more one is going to sit glued to the set and generate a self-induced bombardment of stimulation. Our entrepreneurial masters, moreover, not excessively biblical in their day-to-day living, nevertheless fervently embrace biblical principles when it comes to child development: 'Train up a child in the way he should go, and when he is old, he will not depart from it.'

One is forced, then, not only to confront an immense range of options (so that the prospect of buying a new motor vehicle, for example, opens up an absurdly complex range of possibilities, to the point of inducing anxiety in the most bovine of us), but one is also made to feel substandard and of inferior clay if one is not always making choices. And of course it is not only in the area of consumer goods that this conflict arises — the variety of career choices now available to youth, of both sexes, has made the selection of the correct path much more important than it ever was, for lateral career choices now are small indeed and the penalties for an incorrect choice may go on for life. Even in the spheres of morality and personal behaviour there is now, allegedly for the better, an almost infinite variety of choices of an 'alternative lifestyle'.

Does all this matter, or is it just part of the good fun

of living in an absurdly affluent society? There is certainly some evidence to suggest that it does matter; evidence which links such conflicts, particularly for the more disadvantaged segments of the population, with some forms of delinquency, with urban revolt, with increase in the prevalence of neurotic symptoms. There is evidence, for example, to suggest that the increasing neurotic symptomatology manifested by individuals who move from an African tribal milieu to a coastal city is at least in part due to the dramatic increase in the choices suddenly made available to them, and the pressure to make a choice from seemingly conflicting, often mutually exclusive lifestyles. Industrial psychologists, in their own empirical studies, have suggested that the human organism has only a limited capacity to make choices, and that overload may lead to pathological symptoms such as irritability, disorientation, violent behaviour and psychosomatic illness. This may be part of a general condition of 'input overload', but it is no less relevant for that. Indeed Stanley Milgram, in his classic paper 'The Experience of Living in Cities', has described urban life as consisting of 'a continuous set of encounters with overload'.

While there is money to be made in forcing people to decide whether they want their washing powder to contain fourteen percent of 'blue protocol', or whether they will opt for a rival product which is seventeen percent whiter (whiter than what? — as Stan Freberg used to say), then presumably there is no specific remedy that we can foreshadow for this particularly disastrous effluent from an affluent society. One is even asked to make a decision as to how one intends to satisfy a need one didn't know one had! — so that much of the anxiety of the immediate future may be anxiety derived from an artificial provocation of greed. The analyst

Helm Stierlin puts it this way: '...a revolution of desires, a hunger for constantly stimulated consumption ...a search for pleasure or happiness which is bound to become only more intense and restless as the means to achieve it seem to become legion.'

It would be idle therefore to pretend that we are dealing with anything other than a state of virtually continuous, non-physiological arousal in a variety of somatic systems, as one consequence of today's technological society — and an arousal which the standard mental defence mechanisms are virtually powerless to modulate. And one may predict, I fear, that this situation is going to get worse before it gets better. After all, we live in a society which, whether it is talking about noise, armaments, sex or motor cars, only survives on the enthusiastic assumption that 'more is better'. Oscar Wilde had an epigram for it: 'Nothing succeeds like excess'.

It is scarcely revolutionary to point out the consequences for modern man of the increasing urbanization and industrialization of a rapidly widening segment of the world's population. Durkheim was concerned about this almost a century ago, and countless philosophers, psychiatrists and political scientists have agonized since that time about the impact on mankind of the growth of technology and automation and the consequent decrease, often almost to vanishing point, in the creative satisfaction involved in earning one's living. Fragmentation of the industrial process, the dehumanization inherent in the assembly line approach to production — these things are not conducive to a comfortable, positive self-image. One of the major problems of our society in the future involves what to do for the proportion of the population whose image of itself is loaded with a pervasive sense of failure and insignificance. The resulting impoverishment in self-esteem (if indeed it ever existed for many of these children and adults) is incompatible with a non-anxious, relaxed acceptance of oneself and one's life. It is idle to pretend that the rapid growth in social services and other benevolent protective devices can do anything very much to modify such self-defeating downward spirals; this development in the evolution of our society is more truly a symptom of our malaise, rather than an effective treatment for it. (Which is not of course to infer that we should cease providing such protection.)

What Stainbrook has called 'the anonymous and therefore casual and uncommitted relationship to neighbourhood and community' is probably, however, a much more significant aspect of modern life, as far as the generation and in particular the containment of anxiety are concerned. Even though, as I have stated earlier, the fundamental roots of anxiety are not to be found in contemporary social experience, however catastrophic, there is by now good evidence that the social network in which an individual is embedded will be of critical importance in determining whether that person is troubled by anxiety symptoms, whether he will disintegrate under acute stress, or whether he is able to manage his intrapsychic and interpersonal conflicts without significant disturbance of his lifestyle or sense of comfort. There is by now a good deal of experimental evidence, notably in Leighton's Stirling County study, that the mental health of a community will be improved where the community can be more effectively integrated, and social psychologists have shown us that an individual's level of psychological distress can be inversely correlated with the support that he perceives within his own social network. We need not idealize the concept of community, yet we must acknowledge that the decline of organized religion, the eclipse of national pride, and the media's incessant debunking, in a new version of Totem and Tabu, which has made less possible an uncritical adoration of national heroes — all have taken away some of the sources of identity and belonging for many of those individuals whose psychopathological conflicts made it difficult or impossible for them to achieve or maintain real self-esteem without a heavy reliance on these now absent sources of group solidarity.

In the big city the individual tends, as Milgram has emphasized, to lack a sense of direct contact and integration with the life around him; he needs the institutions which are inseparable from city life to protect him from some of its more difficult aspects, yet these same institutions, interposed between him and his world, estrange him from that world in a functionally dislocating manner. There is much to suggest that self-esteem, the best of all antidotes to anxiety, can be greatly enhanced or maintained by the sense of belonging to a small community or social group, particularly where the group itself has an esteem which 'rubs off' on its members. In these detribalized times, it seems to have become increasingly uncommon for individuals to derive strength from a sense of community, in its most important meaning, that of 'feeling of belonging together', an awareness of common interest and some sense of shared past and shared future. A feeling of alienation, deep psychological roots though it may well have, is greatly magnified in such a climate — and alienation means anxiety, or else elaborate defences against it.

Recently the International Red Cross, in collaboration with a Swiss pharmaceutical company, sponsored a publication entitled 'Health in 1980-1990'. Many distinguished psychiatrists, physicians and social scientists participated in this exercise in futurology, including several from Australia. One or two quotations from this fascinating publication may help you to see that I am not alone in my somewhat pessimistic view of tomorrow's society: they say, for instance, 'short of a radical and purposeful re-structuring of society, which seems highly improbable at least in this century, man will show increasing failure to adapt to his environment. This process of decompensation is at the root of the prodigious rise in neurotic illness.' They believe that this tremendous increase in neurosis will stimulate the search for new psychotropic drugs, apparently giving up in despair when they contemplate the possibility of correcting the psychosocial factors in tomorrow's environment; they display, however, a greater faith than my faithless soul allows me when they predict that the development of psychopharmacology will mean that 'all types of neuroses will become treatable and perhaps curable'. (Are they inferring that we will be able to cure neuroses regardless of any environmental issues at all? — they seem in fact to withdraw from this extreme view in a later chapter.)

To my mind, the matter is rather more complicated than this. I have no doubt that the currently available anxiolytic drugs, plus those that will succeed them, will remain extremely valuable weapons in our therapeutic armamentarium when anxiety symptoms are overt and disabling; but they will never represent, as Leo Hollister puts it, '...more than symptomatic adjunctive treatment'. (In the same paper Hollister points out that 'unless physicians learn to use these drugs with restraint, political pressures stemming from the growing problem of drug abuse may lead to unwise constraints, a view which, interestingly enough, is shared by the futurologists to whom I have just referred, who feel that 'public reaction against psychotropic drugs will be strengthened by a growing realization that many of their apparent benefits are illusory, and that their use is a confession of failure by the individual and by society'.)

Much of the difficulty is a semantic one, as is so frequently the case when human affects are under consideration. We talk about anxiety as if it were, by definition, a pathological state, totally ignoring the existential view that anxiety is an essential experience for any man who is oriented towards freedom. The existentialists maintain, indeed, that in running away from anxiety the individual is likely to lose a uniquely valuable opportunity for education as a human being. The futurologists say much the same thing when they point out that 'the chemical screen may merely provide a transient escape from problems of social integration or of personal relationships, but there is the danger that it may put off forever the finding of true solutions to these problems.' My New Zealand colleague Reg Medlicott, one time President of the College of Psychiatrists, has made a useful distinction between 'anxiety' (as a morbid condition) and what he calls 'anxious dissatisfaction...the anxiety of living'. Like many of us, he is concerned by the growth of what he calls the 'ataractic philosophy whereby suffering or displeasure whether anxiety, depression or pain are viewed as entirely negative states which must be relieved or eradicated on sight'. Doctors do not like the feeling of anxiety any more than anyone else does — they may even like it less, though paradoxically it would appear that they probably experience more than their fair share; it is devoutly to be wished, nevertheless, that in the management of his own affective states, as well as those of his patients, the physician will attempt to differentiate along lines similar to those employed by Medlicott so that, when it is clear that he is dealing with anxious dissatisfaction rather than pathological anxiety, he can encourage his patient (or himself) 'to move through the anxiety-producing situation rather than avoid it'.

Tension: the Basis of Psychosomatic Disease

Dr Alec Dempster

LOOKING INTO THE little minute to minute details of our daily thoughts and actions the manifestations of our tensions appear ubiquitous. Hidden from sight and consciousness in each of us are so many memories, habitual tendencies and forces, but most people recognize very few of these.

While falling asleep many have experienced a sudden violent, brief jerk of their body which was involuntary and without forewarning. All of us when trying to concentrate, have found our thoughts wandering far from the intended path. Some cannot slow their thoughts enough to go to sleep until hours have passed. Obviously examples of tension, these experiences reflect the 'inside pressures' in us.

Most of us live in a constant state of tension. It is deeply woven into our psychological make-up, and we see only its most superficial appearances. Not having much experience of freedom from our own internal strains and blockages, reminds one of a disturbed person who is trying to imagine what he would be like if he was mentally healthy. Although he vaguely knows his predicament, he cannot free his imagination from bizarre distortions. Literally speaking, tension from the health point of view is an insane way of living. For the most of us our whole being is charged with tension. In observing the occurence of our thoughts we realize our subconscious mind is the primary repository, but our personalities and life-style exude it: we carry an 'air of tension' wherever we go. Just as we do not usually see the gaseous air around us, the air of personality we project is often invisible to its owner, as he or she grossly misperceives himself or herself.

An air of personality which is thick with tension has vivid effects on others. Although just as real in its effects, a minor degree of tension in others is usually detected only by our subconscious mind, for we are usually otherwise consciously preoccupied.

A young man recently was in a severe state of anxiety which had developed over the past two years. Each day he was gripped, without warning by attacks of panic. His thoughts would begin to race, a sense of fear of impending death overtook him, and his heart would race and palpitate. A choking sensation closed in on his chest and with his response of desperate rapid breathing would come numbness and temporary paralysis. Sitting quietly in the presence of this man was like being near a high voltage generator. The intense fear and nervous overactivity had a high potential for shaking up anyone else with him. Yet notwithstanding this, he could not see his problem as definitely that of tension, but wondered whether it was a heart condition until further discussion helped bring out his underlying personal problems.

It is not my purpose here to academically categorize tensions, and it is doubtful whether the psychiatric 'diagnostic pigeonholes' provide a satisfactory basis for understanding these factors in operation in the mind. The notion of tension is not generally seen as a 'clearly definable separate entity'. Possibly tension, in medical thinking, seems an ill-defined, unsophisticated, global term. But modern psychology and psychiatry embrace a wide variety of differing opinions on valid classifications and terminology. Furthermore, its commonness in everyday language and thought give it very practical usefulness and justification.

We must go beyond the 'illness' categories of medical thought and look at the emotional reactions and activities of everyday life. Here many of us are displaying little symptoms and habits which psychiatry could consider perfectly normal and healthy because it identifies commonness and the average as normal. (This is a viewpoint which has been derived from philosophy. Kierkegaard described two types of anxiety — 'normal anxiety' of daily life, and 'neurotic anxiety' which he postulated came from the dread of non-existence) (1) Yet these symptoms and habits are the basis of psychosomatic disorders.

We can easily see simple factors in tension. Conditioning is important. By repetition of daily disturbances the habit of being disturbed is developed. Through practice, wrong attitudes such as impatience, carelessness and their resulting tensions become built into us as a more permanent feature. This conditioning process is deliberately used in psychological methods. But most of us have unwittingly and very successfully trained ourselves to be tense through habitually adopting attitudes of discontent, jealousy, ambition, impatience and so on.

Tension means conflict. We want to be natural and have knowledge, freedom and peace. But in our ignorance, we have adopted a set of underlying beliefs, assumptions, attitudes and values — a personal philosophy which is often more subconscious than deliberate and which inevitably leads us into situations and experiences which conflict with what is more fundamentally right.

For clarity we may refer to two levels of tension — external and internal. The external subjectively felt tensions are feelings of uneasiness and physical disturbance usually intermittently apparent to us. However the internal component is present continuously in our subconscious psychology and is always exerting its influence. The manifestations of this are recognized with the development of greater self-awareness, for instance, the parent who bursts out with real anger when disciplining a child, but who describes it as necessary guidance, ignoring the destructive release of his or her own anger, may be helped to recognize this anger and, if need be, adopt a different approach.

Tension of course refers not only to anger and anxiety but to all the negative emotional reactions and their physical manifestations. The symptoms of anxiety are well-known, including those we have already described and others such as weakness, trembling hands, urgency to urinate, diarrhoea, sweating, skin pallor and worried looks. That physiological and biochemical disturbances closely correlate with emotional reactions is well-known. Prolonged tensions thereby lead to dysfunction, bodily and personality deterioration, and gross psychosomatic disease. It is said that the patterns of decay and disease are partly determined by weaknesses which the body has previously acquired or inherited. A large number of psychosomatic organic disease states are now recognized.

The first stage of the psychosomatic process may not usually be noticed by us because of lack of self-awareness, and our ignorance of principles, techniques and standards of daily care of the body. This is an important point. Contemporary Western medicine has not recognized how little understanding it has to offer, how primitive and few are its techniques for proper servicing or maintenance of the body, not to mention health care of the mind. In this regard — the preventive approach — Western medicine pales into insignificance in comparison with the authoritative, sophisticated knowledge available from other sources, such as Yoga and related methods of self-development.

Tension is generally poorly dealt with. Escapes are often found in harmful outlets such as excess alcohol, overworking and so on. Myths are very prevalent. We can explain it away as the result of outside influences — our job, the pace of life etc. — instead of admitting that it is a result of our inability to live in ways which would enable us to cope with these influences. Some believe they need tension because it drives them to greater success. They would do well to examine the quality and permanence of their success. Others say 'you cannot change yourself so you are stuck with tension' which is a naive and unfortunate psychological theory.

Relaxation is the antithesis of tension. A booming interest in it reflects the prevalence of stress today. Of course commercial exploitation and quackery abound. Sensational distractions for the mind provide temporary abatement, but an increase of problems afterwards. Biofeedback and muscular relaxation techniques may offer a little through superficial experiences. Various psychotherapies may help, as well as psychoactive drugs in crises. Another approach — 'doing your own thing' — is good when it means a period of relaxation. But when it means the person's formula for freedom is neglect of moral principles, responsibility and social laws — a rejection of self-control — then this leads directly to greater unhappiness. And this is done because fundamental principles are not understood.

The first fundament of relaxation is concentration. This is the secret of relaxation. Using techniques whereby other things are shut out, the conscious distractions and drifting thoughts temporarily gone, an equipoise ensues. Without mental interference, the body functions naturally and we can work effectively in a calm state of single-mindedness.

To develop this capacity requires a disciplined effort, and gradual learning from the resulting experiences. By following this path unhelpful habits, motivations, attitudes and weaknesses are found blocking the way. Gradually surmounting these brings a growth of self-awareness. The elimination of tensions which are now more clearly seen means you will become a more relaxed person.

Total character development is the authentic synonym of true relaxation. Every facet of our person waits to be examined, understood and corrected to enable as complete an elimination of tension as possible. It takes time, perseverance, willingness to suffer humiliation and pain, but eventually it releases greater contentment, happiness and a greater feeling of freedom. How often have we, in our hearts, yearned for freedom and for our burdens to go away? By overcoming tension we become happier in ourselves, are free to enjoy life more, and more free to serve others. We can develop from our mundane mentality caught up in little every-day problems to a more profound experience of life.

1. Sim, M. 'Guide to Psychiatry', E.&S. Livingston., London (1969).

Emotional Education

Dr Satya Pal Duggal

LIFE IS A SERIES of experiences, pleasant as well as unpleasant, but continuous and interconnected. An experience may be analysed into knowing or awareness of the external stimulus; feeling or changes within the organism that decide the nature and intensity of action and prepare the organism for action; and response. When the preparatory stage is conspicuous because of the demands of the situation, it is called emotion. All the emotions except depression make the heart, lungs and ductless glands work faster than their normal rate of work and the activity of the stomach and intestines is suspended. It indirectly indicates that the organism is unprepared or incompetent to meet the situation. Thus consumption of energy proceeds rapidly while the process of assimilaation is stopped, with the result that reserves of energy are also put to use. Harmony of the forces working within the organism usually remains disturbed and the organism lives under strain.

Constant strain or intense strain may damage the biological system considerably and affect the efficiency in normal dealings of life. Therefore, it is of vital importance to the individual and to the society to take care of these emotional forces as early as possible. Ability to regulate and control feelings may be termed emotional education. It should enable the individual to determine the nature and intensity of response in such a way that he or she is no longer a slave of the stimuli but master, and is able to use them for the evolution of the personal and social self.

Modern psychologists recognize that man has no set way of responding to the instructive stimuli. He has to learn every response, because he can learn an infinite variety of responses.

Secondly, man is a habit-forming animal. Once he learns to derive pleasure through an act, he tends to repeat it and in due course it becomes a strong need.

Thirdly, emotions become a force when they are stimulated i.e. on the perception of a stimulus. In fact, stimulus becomes a stimulus only when it is perceived as such. By consciously attending to some other activity and ignoring the stimulus, excitement may be delayed or even postponed.

Fourthly, frequent stimulation of one emotion or the other, and an exciting atmosphere, are the characteristics of modern civilization. The rush of life due to the struggle for more and more material comforts further accentuates this trend.

Fifthly, reduced vitality whether because of fatigue, illness, worry etc. makes the organism more susceptible to emotional reaction.

Some people argue that present day life is full of strains and the best method to prepare us to bear those strains is to live under strain so that we may become habituated to them. But this way of thinking is based on faulty assumptions. Why after all should one bear strain? Is it an end in itself? Certainly not. Health may be accepted as the desirable objective. Health is a state of the organism that finds manifestation in the feeling of harmony, efficiency in work, an ability to meet an emergent situation calmly, to arrive at appropriate decisions quickly and above all, longevity. Habituation to emotional excitement reduces vitality, impairs health considerably, and decreases the ability to bear the strains of life. Life under normal conditions i.e. without deviations equips one better to face future emergencies.

An eminent British psychologist, Cyril Burt, is of the view that deflection and substitution may result in partial sublimation, but the deflection of the specific energy of the particular instinct, say sex, would be much more doubtful. Burt therefore, would suggest periodical stimulation and satisfaction of various tendencies.

Psychoanalysts emphasize that dissatisfied urges become part of the unconscious and demand satisfaction in future, either directly, or in the form of an abnormal pattern of behaviour. Contemplated action activates the muscles immediately. If there is no overt action, tension persists in the muscles. Psychoanalysts advise us to follow the path of least resistance by providing for the satisfaction of each emotion that is aroused.

These two approaches recognize that supremacy of the exciting stimuli. The idea that impulses can be and should be controlled at the emotional level is ignored.

Catharsis of emotional reactions in the form of games, drama, painting, creative writing etc. makes emotional forces ineffective to some extent. But the medium of catharsis may not be available all the time and tension may persist till the action is executed. Modern psychology has nothing better to offer in this regard.

But recognizing the intimate relationship between the body and the mind, it is proper to expect the possibility of controlling and regulating emotional reactions through some form of psycho-physical education. A healthy body is the sine qua non of emotional education. Prevalent systems of physical education lay emphasis on muscles, and generally ignore the nervous system. Moreover these involve emotional excitement in the form of competition. Consequently there is little refinement of emotions through them.

Essential factors for emotional education are:

(a) A balanced philosophy of life leading to a detached and objective outlook thus eliminating worry.

(b) Concentration leading to planned perception and conscious action.

(c) Balanced exercise of all the organs to ensure normal functioning and to test their vitality to meet demands of emergency.

(d) Relaxation to release muscular and nervous tension.

To accomplish this we must become habituated to a moral way of life. For this, contemplation is the only available technique. It involves interpretation of life and its purpose. Moral values are fitted in the matrix of life. Repeated resolve to lead a life shaped along these lines and constant evaluation of one's conduct in the light of this resolve change one's very personality and perspective on life. One becomes the creator of one's environment and no longer a straw blown about by the wind of circumstances. Yoga emotional education is based on these solid, moral foundations.

Additionally Yoga embraces postural training (asana) and control of the bioenergy (pranayama) which improve the vitality of the system as a whole and are conducive to emotional stability. Yoga physical education is unique in so far as it is non-fatiguing, non-violent and involves a minimum consumption of energy. It is remedial as well as preventive. Bioenergy control (pranayama), abstraction (pratyahara) and concentration (dharana) are methods of bringing the restless thought process under conscious control. Regulated perception coupled with periodical conscious and complete relaxation make emotional disturbances rare in the life of a sincere student of Yoga.

These practices help to make life rhythmic and harmonious. The only price one has to pay for them is the patience to continue practising them.

On Psychosomatic Disease

Dr John Pawsey

A WORKING DEFINITION of psychosomatic can be derived from a breakdown of the word; 'psyche' being taken as the conscious and unconscious process of storage of sensory data, retrieval of memories, and the synthesis, from these past and present components, of current thoughts and attitudes. 'Soma' has the usual meaning of anatomical body and its physiological functions. Disease can be thought of as occurring when some physiological activity is changed sufficiently to make the life of the individual uncomfortable.

Such changes can arise in all aspects of physiological activity, from the rapid dilation of the small blood vessels in the skin when blushing from embarassment to nervous gastro-intestinal symptoms.

Because diseases are generally the result of longstanding processes within the body, treatment often needs to be lengthy also. The first requirement is for the individual to regain mental and physical calm thus reducing the overt symptoms. Success at this level encourages the patient to continue association with the therapist. To this end many and various techniques have been evolved and are used by various disciplines of health-practice in all parts of the world. Many appear to have common features, namely repetitive sounds such as chanting of sacred texts or other special words, rhythmic movements of the body and limbs, or concentration on a breathing rhythm, all of which lead to a lulling of the mind thus permitting quietude. Other techniques include concentration on the body and its internal rhythms, thereby relaxing the mind and isolating it from distracting sensations; deliberate application of hypnosis is sometimes used wherein the regular, gentle, repetitive suggestions of relaxation made by the therapist encourage the patient to isolate mind and body from worrying external and internal stimuli. The pharmaceutical agents employed by Western trained medical practitioners, while very useful in controlling the overt symptoms, unfortunately fall far short of being curative; their main role may be that of helping to establish rapport between patient and therapist. Indeed because they can cloud mental processes they can hinder long term re-educational lines of treatment.

From a practical point of view one-for-one therapy may not be possible but satisfactory results can often be achieved in small groups of patients with a therapist. For example, when the form of treatment involves instruction in and practising of regular rhythmic bodily movements and/or special breathing routines, the encouragement from membership of such a therapy group is quite strengthening. It helps the individual to persevere with treatment, especially if it is reinforced by some selective personal attention.

It is common experience that initial gains can be lost if the patient returns to the environmental situation with unchanged attitudes of mind. So, after the initial control of physical symptoms is achieved, therapy should become more oriented to improving the general well-being and strengthening the character of the whole person. It is in this aspect of therapy that Western medicine is deficient and has much to learn; hopefully this will come from observing the success of existing health disciplines from other parts of the world. To accomplish such character building it is desirable for the patient to obtain some understanding of the mechanisms which have been operative over the previous years, not only those which directly led to the disease for which treatment had been sought, but also for all the components upon which the individual's judgement-forming capacity had been based. The individual is encouraged to consciously, and unconsciously, retrieve and reappraise his stored memories, affects and impressions.

Because this process is necessarily accompanied by a great deal of stirring up of anxiety, with the ensuing physical symptoms, the therapist must keep emphasizing the need to maintain a schedule of practices designed to ensure quietude of mind and body. Again, group practices can be very helpful, enabling the individual to go through such a discipline encouraged by an almost unconscious awareness of the well-meaning presence of fellow patients and therapist. This does not, however, obviate the need for the therapist to set out a programme which is suited to the individual patient's needs and abilities.

The ideal situation arises when the patient comes to appreciate the way in which attitudes and standards are derived from his or her concept of the relationship between self and the rest of the universe. This concept of the relationship between self and the universe is ever-changing, evolving each day under the effect of new experiences. The individual can benefit greatly by being exposed to new ideas and teachings of other people who have learned from their own experience, while yet maintaining performance of those practices which have led to the new-found capacity to sit quietly and digest old and new ideas.

Groups can also participate in discussions based on themes introduced to them by a therapist, or others who have experienced and achieved worthwhile goals in life. It may be that the initial practices need to be modified to match the evolving capacity and needs of the individual. This is best judged by an experienced teacher-practitioner of a healing art who must therefore be a well experienced and evolved person in order to be able to guide patients in their tortuous progress towards health or wholeness.

Because positive results can be attributed to all the philosophies of healing it would be desirable to objectively examine their differing techniques in order to find the common factor. Perhaps these may then be put to adequate scientific appraisal and made more easily accessible to the suffering humanity.

Psychosomatics in Perspective

Aspects of Treatment

Routines: A Basis for Health

Dr Jayadev Yogendra

THE ESTABLISHMENT of routines is very important, not only from the point of view of health, but also because routines put us in a particular mood or state of mind. We may ask, how can external situations and fixed habits contribute to particular thought patterns? This can best be illustrated by the story of two thieves who were unsuccessful and tried to evolve a new strategy for making money. They finally decided that one of them would become a teacher and the other his disciple. They went to a village where one of them put on the correct type of dress and sat down near a water tank to which the villagers came, closed his eyes and pretended to meditate. The other played the part of an extremely devoted disciple, fanning him and keeping the surroundings free from any nuisance and disturbance. They agreed that the teacher would keep his eyes closed and maintain the position as long as possible. And so he kept up the attitude of deep meditation while the disciple praised the prowess of this great teacher to the people who came near. He did a good job and brought many of the villagers to have darshan (a meeting with a holy man) and, as is customary, the person benefitting from such a darshan put money or some other gift before the great 'saint' he had come to visit.

The disciple was able to encourage many people to come and have darshan and they left a great deal of money. The sound of the money collecting before him encouraged the teacher to maintain his silence and his posture with composure, and to keep his eyes closed. By evening the disciple thought they had earned enough money in an honourable way and felt it was time to go. When nobody was present he tapped the teacher on the shoulder and said: 'We have made enough now. We can think about moving away.' The teacher opened his eyes for the first time and replied: 'I have come to like this. I am not going to go!' A sudden transformation had taken place. This story illustrates how certain habits and routines have a great capacity to make changes within us. If we keep on following positive habit patterns they will ultimately make us better than we were.

We only need a few tools to better ourselves or improve ourselves. We don't have to do hundreds of physical exercises but rather put our faith in very simple occupations like making a study of our motives, keeping a diary, being more mindful of what we are doing, and observing a certain amount of discipline. By such aids a person attempts to maintain correct routines. In India, for instance, a spiritual seeker will start off his day very meaningfully so that he builds up positive habits which in time help him to build up a new state of consciousness.

The person interested in his own development should make a study of his routines and see whether they have been sensibly planned or not. Very often we are not aware of our routines. Many people come to us with lots of problems, some of them health problems; in these cases I make a point of discussing with them what routines they observe, because I believe that diseases are just the result of our wrong habits of living. We are responsible ourselves for our disease conditions, but the problem is to know what we did that led to a disease. I ask people to tell me more about how they spend their day, what they do when they get up and things like that. Sometimes I am surprised how unaware they are of their own day-to-day life. They might report they got up at 5 am, and then the only other thing they could think of would be having a mouthwash, attending the toilet, reading the newspaper, having their breakfast and going to the office. It may be that they got up at five and left at ten. In those five hours they don't know what they did, except for a few things. If one pursues the question they admit that their activities took a total of half an hour or forty five minutes. The rest of the time they do not know what they did. We have no real control over the various things we do regularly.

As far as food habits are concerned the individual must organize his routines so that they continuously contribute to his progress towards his goal. He cannot follow bad routines and expect to achieve a high goal. When it comes to food the ancient yogis maintained that food was a very important means of controlling ourselves. A story from the Upanishads points out that food is Brahman — the very highest reality in this universe, the highest consciousness. The injunction is that food is itself the highest reality and this is illustrated in a beautiful way. A little boy who suddenly thought of gaining spiritual consciousness went up to his teacher and told him: 'I want to develop spiritually.' His teacher looked at the boy and replied: 'Very well, you must fast for one day.' The boy was sincere and did as he was told. He came the next day and said to his teacher: 'I've fasted for one day, now tell me about the highest spiritual consciousness.' The teacher again looked at him and replied: 'No, you must fast for another day.' This went on for another seven days. Every time the boy came up to him the teacher would say: 'No, fast for another day.' On the eighth day the boy didn't turn up so the teacher was a little concerned. He asked the other students what happened and was told that the boy seemed a little weak. The teacher and other students went over to the home of the student and were told that he had not been taking food for several days and was weak lying in bed. They all sat around him and the teacher put the question to the boy: 'My boy, what is Brahman? What is the highest spiritual consciousness?' The boy replied: 'Sir, at the moment I can think of nothing but food.' At that the teacher told him: 'Food is Brahman, food is also a very important ingredient of life.'

This story illustrates that at particular periods of life one has to grow and develop, at others one has to think of spiritual development. It all comes in its own time; one must not neglect any one aspect. Food itself has a tremendous bearing. In fact, if we organize our food habits it can contribute a lot to our spiritual development. In India we think of food in different ways. We don't really think of its protein content or calorific value. We think of its impact on our levels of consciousness. The ancient Indians organized their food habits. The manner in which the food was taken was important: there were specific instructions as to how much food should be taken, at what hours it should be taken, what type of activity should be carried on before and after eating, how the food should actually be consumed. It may seem very strange to us that yogis and spiritual men attended to these matters in such detail. But then the question was: 'Can we divorce any aspect of our life from the highest? or are not all aspects interconnected?'

In the city of Bombay lives a very spiritually developed person. One day someone approached him in the afternoon when he was preparing his food. Knocking at the door at this wrong hour the man said: 'Sir, I want to learn about spirituality.' The other must have been annoyed but didn't show it and replied: 'Very well, we will discuss spirituality. But at the moment, I want some vegetables. I will give you a little money to buy me some.' The man was surprised but accepted the money and went over to the market and bought some vegetables. The holy man told him to prepare and cook them, after which they partook of the food. The wise man then asked the stranger: 'What was it you came for?', to which he replied: 'I came for spiritual learning and you seem to have put me off.' He was told: 'Very well, what we did was on spiritual learning. Your going to the market, getting the vegetables, preparing and cooking the food and our eating the food was all spiritual learning. How do you separate these things? Don't we have to have meals, don't food habits also affect our thinking?' He wanted to bring home the point that nothing we do can be considered as being apart from that which we have set ourselves to do. There are individuals who live for food; most of the time they are thinking of their next meal. They are sometimes so carried away as to eat more than they should and become sick or often they develop perverted tastes. We know how many people today live in this way but this does not contribute to the best kind of development. Food has its own small place and we have to create the right type of habits in this connection. The yogis, for example, eat food four times a day at intervals of about four hours. The food is of a very simple type: no fried things, no spices, no high protein or non-vegetable food and no alcohol of any sort. This is a sort of discipline; not that they do not enjoy it, but they know that if they allow their eating habits free rein, they would live for eating and nothing else would be important to them. Controlling the eating habit also becomes a means of controlling the mind or organizing one's whole life.

In this fashion we can think of various routines throughout the whole day. One can think in terms of relaxation also, and recreation. After all, work is not the only activity in life; one must change from one activity to another. The ancient yogis lived in very beautiful spots: river banks, valleys, mountain-tops and so on; they used to spend part of their time in gardening or just moving around. All work was stopped as soon as the sun set.

These are some of the routines that are followed in India. I do not recommend that all such routines should be followed today, but following some routines has great value because without much effort they can put us in a positive state of mind. When we consider the question of food, for example, and observe a certain amount of control, it helps develop a state of mind in which, in spite of that desire to eat more, or that desire to eat a particular thing, the mind is controlled. In this way we are reminded that we do not live for this one thing, that there is a lot more to us. Once this type of thought process is begun and such thoughts cultivated every day we can develop a certain amount of self-control.

The establishment of certain routines, certain fixed habits, depends on the individual, the availability of time, the nature of his work and so on. However, in spite of the amount of work that one might have, it should be possible to organize definite periods which remind us of the need to change. In India some people spend three times a day in a sort of prayer, and that itself is Yoga. They sit in a particular posture and do certain breathing practices and are very concentrated.

In this way particular attitudes to life are built up. They may look like simple, meaningless, ritual activities but they can also have a lot of meaning. If one does not believe in these sorts of activities, a simple quietening practice can help. One can sit, cut off from outside disturbances, become quietened, take stock of things and try to rededicate oneself to a higher purpose. The type of routine can vary from person to person, from country to country, according to the different situations and can contribute greatly to the maintenance of our health and our capacity to understand ourselves.

Psychosomatic Techniques of Yoga

Dr David Mander and Patrick Dugan

IN YOGA, HEALTH is considered more than just the absence of disease. It is seen as a positive, radiant vitality — a complete harmony of body and mind.

Any deviation from this state of health could be considered ill-health or disease. A large and increasing proportion of such illnesses in contemporary society is now recognized as being psychosomatic in nature. This term applies to a condition of physical discomfort and/or degeneration arising as a result of mental or emotional disturbance. For the purpose of this article, however, the use of the adjective 'psychosomatic' refers to those states of ill-health caused by wrong mental attitudes; or where a change in attitude could result in an almost immediate improvement if not disappearance of the complaint.

In treating problems of ill-health Western medicine relies heavily on two therapeutic techniques — drug treatment and surgery. Thus the patient with a gastric ulcer has the offending tissue removed, while the victim of psychogenic asthma receives bronchodilators to remedy nature's shortcomings. In approaching his patient, the physician sees the body's imperfections as the problem and the chemical creations of the drug houses as the answers. There is seldom the recognition that the body itself contains adequate mechanisms to cope with disease, nor the understanding of the conditions necessary for these same mechanisms to operate efficiently.

Understanding diseases arising from wrong mental attitudes requires an understanding of how wrong attitudes develop. Psychiatrists often remark that the human personality is determined in the first two years of life. Whether or not this true, it is apparent that the emotional stability of the mother or lack of it will affect the child in some way, although these effects will not manifest themselves until very much later. For example, an overly-protective mother may instil a sense of fear and lack of initiative into her child; or a parent, insecure himself, may become over-critical and subject a child to a continual barrage of criticism, leaving the child with two alternatives: either to withdraw into himself or to become aggressive and fight back. His nature from birth probably determines which alternative he takes; but in either case he develops a negative self-image and a constant fear of failure.

By the time a person reaches early adulthood he has developed what might be termed 'dispositions of behaviour'; he could be disposed to anger, anxiety, or fear, or on the other hand he could be disposed to more positive behaviour. Whichever is the case, as the practice of a particular type of behaviour continues, the disposition hardens to become a habit.

The negative dispositions or attitudes are the forerunners of psychosomatic complaints. The emotion of fear, for instance, produces different reactions in different people but its general effect can be observed in the example of an animal. When an animal is frightened adrenalin is immediately released into the blood and manifests in the 'fight or flight' reaction, either in fighting its enemy or fleeing to safety. After vanquishing the enemy or reaching safety, the fear in the animal subsides, the action having used the extra energy released by the adrenalin. In man, however, this does not occur. His fear or anxiety is a constant, nagging one. He has instinctive reactions similar to those of the animal but these do not cease when the danger is over but continue — for fear has become a habit. In such cases the constant irritation of the bowels can produce colitis, or the adrenalin produced by the tension and unused in action, will cause some serious damage. When the body is put under such continual stress and strain, it will be the weakest of the systems — the weakest link in the chain — which will break down. It is for this reason that generalization is never possible and each case must be looked at individually. Fear will produce psoriasis in one man, asthma in another and colitis in yet another.

Notwithstanding the attention given to the physical body, sound health will not be achieved while the mind is dominated by emotional conflict and tension. Elucidation of the cause of a psychosomatic complaint will be the first step in eliminating it. As mentioned previously some psychosomatic conditions result from anxiety and fear, others result from guilts arising out of actions committed in the past, pressure of life in industrial society, lack of a consistent set of values, attachment to material objects, indiscipline, lack of emotional control, ignorance of the effects of negative thinking and lack of self-awareness. Subconscious fears resulting from unpleasant or traumatic experiences which have occurred at an early age and subsequently been repressed may cause psychosomatic conditions; or else they may be created by the subconscious mind as a means for attracting attention or escaping responsibility.

However, knowledge of the cause is not sufficient in itself. The individual will then have to make a disciplined effort to alter patterns of behaviour established over many years and undergo a fundamental readjustment of his basic attitudes and values. He may have to learn the art of self-observation in order to gain a greater awareness of his own physical and emotional reactions. Thus in the final analysis complete cure of psychosomatic disease rests with the patient. The work of the teacher however, is still indispensable and lies in assisting the patient to see and understand the cause of his difficulties and in providing the techniques and encouragement so that he may be able to overcome them. This is how a Yoga teacher works.

However, to be able to understand the situations of those with whom he is confronted, a Yoga teacher must have sound qualifications. He must first and foremost have a thorough subjective understanding of his own mind and body. Through his understanding, he must gain further insight into the workings of the mind and its effects on the physical body in all human types. Secondly, he must have the capacity for intuitive understanding of a person's personality and problems. Thirdly he must have an unfailing positive approach towards his life and work which allows him to inspire a similiar attitude in those whom he serves, and finally, he requires a detailed knowledge of the specific effects of the various Yoga practices.

Some of the techniques a Yoga teacher uses to help someone suffering from a psychosomatic complaint will include asanas — Yoga physical practices — and pranayama — breathing techniques. These have an effect mainly on the nervous system, lungs, endocrine glands, heart and abdominal viscera, rather than on the muscular system, and may have a psychosomatic effect. The slow rhythmic nature of many asanas has a soothing influence on the mind and the techniques of pranayama gradually bring under control irregular breathing patterns and bring about a reduction in the rate of breathing, thereby producing a quieter and more controlled state of mind.

There are two simple techniques in Yoga which can offer a person help in (a) reducing tension already existing in the mind, and (b) developing greater awareness of the sources of tension. Basically, it is the function ing and reactions of the mind that create tension in the body. External situations are merely the triggers which set off the cycle of emotional thinking in the form of worries, resentments, anger, guilt etc. When the mind is quietened, and the level of thinking reduced, the body returns to its natural, relaxed, tension-free state. The ability to quieten their own minds is something people find especially difficult today, but with persistent practice of the following techniques it can be learnt.

The first technique has been called conditioning by Shri Yogendraji, Founder of The Yoga Institute. It is used as a preparatory practice for the physical practices (asanas). Its effect is to quieten the mind enabling a greater mental involvement in the performance of the practices, and a more relaxed state thus making the practices more efficient. It is normally practised in the meditative posture sukhasana or 'easy pose'. In this posture the legs are crossed, the palms placed on the knees, the spine held straight, the head erect and the eyes closed. The mind is quietened by one of a number of methods. The first method is to take the role of an observer of the functioning of the mind. Thoughts are noted as they appear and allowed to pass without further involvement of the mind. There is no attempt to encourage or discourage thoughts but just to maintain an awareness of any mental activity. It is inevitable that at times the mind will become involved in the thoughts themselves and lose the 'awareness'. As soon as this is discovered the mind should be brought back to the task of observing the thoughts but with no feeling of frustration or annoyance at having failed. The second conditioning method is to focus the mind on any physical sensation involved in sitting in the posture. It could be just the total feeling of the posture, or a particular aspect such as the weight of the hands resting on the knees, or the erectness of the spine. Sometimes if the posture is new, some feelings of discomfort in the back and thighs can be noticed, and these themselves can be used as a point of concentration. The third alternative is to attempt to engender a feeling of 'sinking'. This can be achieved by imagining that one is in a lift or in some other situation of imagined descent. As in the first alternative, in the latter two if the mind wanders from its task, it should be brought back objectively and persistently.

The second technique is a practice called Yogendra Nispanda Bhava or listening. A great advantage of this practice is that it can be performed in any place at any time. It is done in any comfortable sitting position which can be maintained without movement for the period of the practice. The mind is allowed to listen to whatever sounds are apparent. It is a technique of passively 'listening' rather than actively hearing sounds. Thoughts, whether connected or unconnected with the sounds, are replaced in the mind by the sounds alone.

In the beginning concentration in either of these techniques may last for periods which make up only a small proportion of the total time spent on the practices in general. Yet this short experience of quietude has a remarkable effect on the state of the mind and the reduction of physical tension.

As well as these techniques the Yoga teacher must recognize that moral doubts or conflicts between the beliefs a person holds and his actual behaviour cause fear and guilt and as a result psychosomatic complaints.

Because of this it is necessary for a person to accept and follow in practice a consistent set of moral and behavioural values. Attachment to the ego, to temporal values, will inevitably be the cause of tension through fear at some stage in a person's life; hence the values and attitudes accepted by the individual must not be those of attachment to material possessions, status or sensual pleasures as such attitudes will always be associated with fears.

In certain psychosomatic conditions, medical treatment through drugs helps to achieve a temporary alleviation of symptoms, while the process of removing the cause, or overcoming the basic weakness continues. However, drugs can never provide a permanent cure for these conditions, hence a person who genuinely desires to overcome his difficulties must seriously apply himself using the methods outlined above. Although he will probably need the help of a teacher, counsellor or therapist, the effort and motivation must ultimately come from the individual himself. Thus the teacher's role is to provide the appropriate techniques, to supervise their practice, to monitor the student's progress, and to provide encouragement and support when needed. Ultimately it will be the patient who cures himself through his increased understanding, awareness and self-discipline.

On Psychosomatic Health Care

Jan Dugan

IT SEEMS THAT THE word 'psychosomatic' is interpreted in many different ways in the community today. One approach implies that a psychosomatic complaint has no organic basis, the pain and symptoms being merely a figment of the person's imagination. I would like to suggest that a psychosomatic illness or problem is a genuine somatic condition which has its origin principally in an unstable and impure mind. I believe that the tremendous complexity and potential power of the human mind must be thoroughly appreciated and respected. In psychosomatic complaints, this power or capacity of the mind has often become channelled or conditioned in a negative way, or is locked up in a fixation on a problem. As I see it, an individual's state of health at any one time is a manifestation of his total functioning as a human being. This would embrace the body, the mind and the spirit — these three elements being inextricably interwoven and interlinked. Even small complaints such as headaches, sore throats, tension, back pain, indigestion and nasal congestion I see as symbolic physical expressions of a lack of contentment, fulfilment and peace of mind.

In its natural state, undisturbed by emotional factors, urges or impulses, the body runs smoothly and harmoniously. However, when we are anxious, resentful, excited or crave something, the mind becomes agitated and in this condition more nervous energy is needed to sustain it. Hence, some of the energy necessary for the functioning of the organs, for the efficient circulation of the blood or for the glandular processes, is depleted. When this happens regularly and habitually, there is a constant interruption to the natural functioning of the various systems of the body. Each person will respond in a different way, but in time, this will eventually lead to a malfunction, impairment or breakdown in one of the systems.

From a therapeutic point of view, it is helpful with psychosomatic problems to look at the total individual — not just at his physical complaints, or his own verbalization of what is wrong, or merely at the mental aspects. It is helpful to look behind the presented problem to the person's lifestyle, to the way he spends his time, and to the attitudes and values which guide his thinking. There is often a need to train the mind, to cultivate a deeper awareness and to gradually weed out the negative facets of our thinking and allow the mind to return to a more peaceful, harmonious state. Such an approach is a long-term process. It could perhaps be seen as a re-education in the techniques of living which foster a more integrated body-mind complex. If we are looking beyond temporary palliatives and makeshift cures, I feel we must be working towards establishing habits of thinking and behaviour which can be the foundation of permanent good health. I would now like to mention some of the approaches and techniques I have found beneficial in psychosomatic healing.

Viewed simply, the factors which have the greatest potential for disturbing and unsettling the mind are the negative impulses and emotions such as fear, guilt, envy resentment, hatred, anger, lust and greed. The propensity for expressing these states of mind has accumulated over a period of time, and so these habits and patterns of thinking have to be slowly replaced with more positive ones. These positive attitudes or values seem to be the foundation stone of a healthy, resilient mind. For example if we take up the principle of honesty in an absolute, unconditional way, guilts, uncertainties and fears can gradually be eliminated; through practising tolerance and patience, anger is reduced and through bringing forgiveness, acceptance and compassion to bear, hatred can be diminished and eventually overcome.

I feel we can never underestimate the potency of these deeply entrenched emotional reactions. I have found that by consistently holding a principle or a value, rather than allowing fear, guilt or any other emotional factor to dominate my thinking, this has gradually brought about a weakening and an atrophy of these emotional states. A list of simple values can serve as strong guidelines for dealing with and overcoming these emotional reactions.

They might include the following:

- Self-acceptance or Self-love: This means fully accepting our limitations and shortcomings while striving to overcome them. Punishing ourselves can only lead to further tension and frustration.
- Practising Contentment: This involves gradually reducing the number of wants and desires and learning to accept situations as they arise. This will aid in bringing about a state of mental equilibrium.
- Developing Patience with ourselves and others: This is really the capacity to enjoy waiting without looking for quick results. To practise this successfully involves living right within the present moment.
- Showing Perseverance: The ability to persist, to

keep going with quiet determination despite repeated set-backs and disappointments. This is an invaluable quality to foster when we are overcoming problems.

These positive values have no capacity in themselves to create anxiety, guilt or tension; for when a person knows he has done nothing wrong, in the sense of harming himself or another, his conscience is clear, and his mind is purified a little. This knowledge will, in time, produce greater mental stability. The absolute nature of these principles and the approach we adopt in practising them is very important. If they are conditional on certain circumstances or moods, we can easily slip into rationalizations, justifications and suit our own convenience. The time will rarely be right for practising something when sacrificing our pleasure and comfort is concerned. Through exercising restraint, self-control and self-discipline, feelings of a deeper respect and confidence in oneself can gradually be earned.

An approach I have found most valuable and which I see as a vital key to emotional stability and prevention of psychosomatic complaints is training the mind to be more concentrated. Techniques of concentration are suitable and therapeutic for even the most distracted mind. If these can be applied in a regular and consistent way, starting off with perhaps ten minutes daily, the mind can over a period of time become habituated to a more peaceful, concentrated state. When the mind is constantly being irritated or unsettled by unwanted thoughts and urges, it never has the chance to rest or be quiet. The various facets of thinking which disturb the mind can be brought to settle by restricting the activity of the mind in a disciplined way. This helps to slow the mind down, to reduce the number of thoughts and thus to lessen general tension and anxiety, affecting both body and mind. By quietening the mind, we are also conserving our energy. There is no loss of energy through the senses and the emotions at that time. The mind ultimately stays contained within. Through the consistent practice of these techniques we can build up a reserve of energy or greater vitality which will serve in times of crisis and emotional upheaval.

As well as the practice of specific techniques of concentration, I have found it helpful to try to bring an attitude of concentration to whatever I do throughout the day. Work or activity has enormous therapeutic potential if our attitude towards it is a positive one. Through involving the mind in a task or job and attempting to concentrate on it, to bring the full capacity of the mind to bear on the task in hand, we can find temporary release from our self-preoccupations and fears. When the mind is fully concentrated in the present moment, we are free from emotionalism and will therefore be more relaxed. The attitude we bring to a task is important also. Mostly when we are involved in work, our main concern is for the outcome, the fruits of our labour. We are always looking for the reward or the compensation. This attitude seems to create emotional instability. If we fail, or fall short of our objective, we may become depressed or apathetic and this inhibits us in our further attempts. On the other hand if we are successful, we can become over-confident and lose a balanced perspective. This makes us less prepared for any future setbacks or rebuffs, and can lead to criticism and intolerance of others who cannot match our standards. So if we can foster an attitude of enjoying work for its own sake, and devoting our best effort to any piece of work, however menial, I feel this will also contribute to a healthier and more settled condition of the mind.

I feel that where there are psychosomatic problems, it

is advisable to keep physically active and involved. In this way the mind has less opportunity to lapse back into its own negative preoccupations. It can be very therapeutic to express ourselves in activities we enjoy and can be creative in. I would always suggest taking up hobbies and recreational pursuits as a positive way of channelling energy and distracting the mind from its worries. This will contribute to a more relaxed frame of mind. Walking in a garden or a park, and allowing oneself to enjoy the stillness of the water or the graceful movements of the birds will have a soothing effect on the nervous system. Similarly listening to quiet music can be an aid to relaxation. When the mind is severely churned up or disturbed, vigorous physical activity can provide a release. It is helpful too to work towards effecting a balance in the day's activities. Greater harmony can be experienced in daily life when we devote some time to work, some time to recreation and pleasure, some time to duties to oneself and some to the duty of meeting the needs of others.

I have found it most valuable to develop the capacity to observe oneself closely in a detached, disinterested way. Through this, we can become aware of the consequences of our thoughts and actions, and this can provide us with the motivation and the direction for change. We can build up a more objective understanding of ourselves without the interference of value judgements or self-condemnation. We can note which factors enhance our vitality, and which factors distract the mind, sap our strength and deplete the energy. As an aid to this process of self-observation, the use of a diary, in the form of a list of questions to be reviewed at the end of each day, has many advantages. The particular questions to be included will vary with each individual, but a sample might include the following:

1. What time did I get up today?

2. How much time did I spend in quiet and reflection today?
3. How many times did I get angry (hurt, upset, resentful, etc.) today?
4. Why? What were the circumstances?
5. What positive qualities am I trying to develop in myself?
6. Did I forgive myself today when I made a mistake, or fell short of my expectations?
7. Did I show patience and tolerance today? When?
8. What negative qualities am I trying to eradicate in myself?
9. Did I serve someone today without looking for a reward?

The diary can provide a form of positive re-conditioning, in that each day we are reminding ourselves, and reinforcing the notion that certain qualities are desirable to develop. It helps to keep uppermost in the conscious mind the areas we are working on for our own self-improvement. In itself, the diary is a discipline, and this can give form and structure to the day and assist in building habits of consistency. Over a period of time, patterns will emerge in our reactions to situations and people. If we can see the trends in our thinking more explicitly, in time this can prevent the constant repetition of similiar situations which are causing suffering. I have always found that any practice or discipline we take up can provide an excellent framework for self-understanding. The diary can help to pinpoint more clearly our particular tendencies, weaknesses or the fluctuations in our moods and attitudes.

A helpful approach with emotional and psychosomatic problems is to try to be outgoing, concerned and involved with other people. Often when we have an unpleasant experience, the tendency is to become withdrawn and unhappy, immersed in ourselves and resentful of calls on our time or energy. Sometimes the mind is churning over the problem, unable to really accept it, and trying to find a reason for the condition. This approach never seems to prove beneficial. More frequently it seems to compound the problem with tension, frustation and a sense of guilt at our total self-absorption. If we hurt people, neglect their needs or overlook them when we are in this frame of mind, we are apt to regret it later. We may create for ourselves more confusion, misunderstanding and complex situations to untangle. So from the therapeutic point of view, I feel that a consistently caring and outgoing attitude to others, despite what we are suffering will help us progress.

Psychosomatic Aspects of Dental Care

Dr Ronald French

THE MOUTH AND FACE have such deep psychological meaning to human beings from infancy to old age that it should present no surprise that they are subject to emotional factors.

The mouth is the first source of bodily pleasure which may be one reason why pain in this area is so especially resented. From childhood on, the mouth is used both as a source of sensory satisfaction, as in sucking, eating or kissing, and also as a weapon of defence such as biting, arguing or attacking with words. The mouth continues to play an important role in expressing sexual desires on the one hand, as well as rage, self-defence and determination on the other. The age-old awareness of body language is shown in such expressions as, 'he gnashed his teeth', or 'he set his jaws in determination'.

Since the mouth is a tender orifice, essential for breathing, eating and swallowing, its immobilization or invasion tends to lead to special feelings of helplessness and panic in many individuals. In adulthood the mouth and face continue to be invested with great emotional significance, not only because of their role in sexual attractiveness but also because a person's sense of himself becomes so identified with his facial appearance. Thus, any changes in the appearance or function of this vital area may have prolonged ramifications beyond the immediate physical facts.

Personality development is closely linked with a person's self-estimation. A stimulating experience in dentistry is to see the improvement in personality and sometimes in physical development when an unsatisfactory dentition is restored or realigned into harmony with the rest of the face. A case of this type involved a young lad aged thirteen years, lacking in self-confidence and light in build who presented with poor dental appearance for which he was the target of uncomplimentary remarks at school. He had very large upper centrals which crossed and the laterals were not present. X-rays revealed poorly developed laterals present that on eruption had not penetrated the tissue. Tips of these teeth were exposed, pins inserted into the teeth and used as a base to build crowns. After the insertion of the crowns the front teeth were able to be straightened orthodontically. There was a most dramatic change in the boy's appearance. There was an even greater change psychologically and physically. His personality developed rapidly as did his physique. Within one year he was Form Captain, doing well at games and was a very happy and well-adjusted boy.

Character development may greatly influence the use of the mouth. The passive dependent individual is apt to develop a childlike, expectant or apathetic facial expression denoting a passive wish to be taken care of. If, as a child, he continued to eat soft foods long past the age when this was normal, his occlusion may even be affected, since chewing hard food is necessary for proper development of jaw muscles. Such individuals are also more susceptible to syndromes such as chronic subluxation of the jaw. On the other hand, the hostile, biting, rigid person may overuse his masticatory muscles and develop habits of bruxism. The teeth may be chronically ground or clenched together, either as a general result of tension or in a specific effort to control the expression of anger.

Prolonged habits of grinding or clenching may have far reaching effects, either by producing irritation to the teeth, the supporting tissues or by producing chronic pain. This latter may lead to a vicious circle where spasm causes pain which in turn leads to more spasm and increased pain, owing to interruption of the normal physiologic patterns where contraction alternates with relaxation. The tense, anxious person with chronically increased tension of jaw muscles is unable to tolerate usual dental procedures without developing excessive spasm and pain. There is increased sensitivity to pain, as though the nervous pathways were already overloaded and could not adequately handle the extra excitation.

Thus there are several different ways in which emotional factors may enhance or actually cause pain. Anxiety may greatly alter the patient's response to organic pain or, on the other hand, anxiety may actually lead him to feel pain without a structural lesion being present.

Pain is an elusive, difficult to define, subjective phenomenon. There is a physical aspect to it and a psychic aspect.

Pain has been described as a multidimensional experience which involves not only the discriminative capacity to identify onset, duration, location and intensity and the physical characteristics of the stimulus, but also includes motivational, emotional and congenital functions leading to avoidance or aversive behaviour.

Pain also involves the private or personal experiences of unpleasantness and the interpretation of the stimulus in terms of present and past events. And of course pain has a strong psychological element and can be entirely psychogenic. A simple definition may be: 'An experience which may result from tissue damage or from the fear of tissue damage or elements of both of these combined'.

The oro-facial area is one of the most complex of regional areas in terms of identification of pain for the following reasons:

1. Facial structures are of diverse embryological origin.
2. They have an extremely complex cranial and cervical innervation and intricate vascular supply.
3. All of the special senses are perceived in the area.
4. The face has special emotional significance arising from its considerable psychological and sociological importance.

Pain arises from:

(a) Teeth and Supporting Structures.

(b) Neighbouring Structures.
  (i) Temporomandibular joint.
  (ii) Salivary glands.
  (iii) Paranasal sinuses.
  (iv) Oral mucous membranes.
  (v) Denture bearing areas.
  (vi) Ears, Tonsils, Eyes.

(c) The Neuralgias.

(d) Vascular Pains. e.g. migraine.

(e) Facial Pain and Habits associated with Psychogenic Component. e.g. atypical facial pain.

(f) Referred Pain.
  (i) From teeth.
  (ii) Sinuses.
  (iii) Other areas. This never crosses the mid-line.

It can be seen from the foregoing discussion that while much dental pain can be clearly identified and causations established, there is still a wide range of conditions where the underlying problem is not of disease origin.

Tension or aggravated problems are wide ranging and vary from the repeated appearance of ulcers in the mouth through to the intolerance to wear dentures.

1. **Apthous Ulcers**: Although small, these cause considerable discomfort and interference with eating. The first sign is a prickly or burning sensation in the mucous membrane which reddens and an ulcer forms within twenty four hours. These ulcers are linked to stress situations and break out in the same individuals periodically after stress.

2. **Neuralgia**: Primary atypical facial neuralgia is also known as hysterical facial pain because no structural lesion seems to be involved. The word neuralgia is used because there are neurologic symptoms without evidence of nerve damage. It is atypical because the pain pattern is inconsistent and varies tremendously from patient to patient. Pain is usually described as chronic or dull. It may persist for years with little change or may vary considerably according to the mood of the patient and the degree of emotional stress. Pain with an organic basis could not persist for such a long period without a demonstrable lesion. Often these patients exhibit other symptoms of anxiety such as insomnia, depression and gastrointestinal complaints.

3. **Temporomandibular Joint pain**: This is a particularly difficult area of dental pain. Clinically there is usually dull pain in the region of the joint and some form of earache. It is made worse with rapid jaw movement, giving sharp pain. Trismus may limit jaw opening. There may be a clicking of the joint and, clinically, wear facets may be seen on the teeth. Sometimes the pain occurs after sleep and disappears during the day.

Dental factors may strongly contribute to this condition, for example lack of posterior teeth allowing insufficient support or imbalance of the bite.

However psychological factors seem more significant. Bruxing, that is grinding or clenching of the teeth, is usually present. This is associated with stress and it is frequent that the bruxing habit occurs during sleep. Spasm of muscles follows and this is the source of the pain rather than the joint itself. This syndrome is an 'emotionally induced psychosomatic disorder'.

Psychiatric study of a large number of cases has shown these patients suffer from a functional disorder, a prolonged, self-perpetuating tensional jaw. It can be likened to the functional low-back pain often resulting from either overstretching or sudden contraction which leads to spasm and pain in a tense person who may feel depressed, overburdened or resentful. A case illustrating this involved a hypertensive lady in her mid fifties who presented with quite severe pain in the right side. She had difficulty eating and the pain was most severe in the morning. Her dental health was excellent. Questioning revealed that her aged mother lived next door and demanded considerable attention. Her husband was a very busy and successful businessman. An overseas trip was taken and she reported that she had no pain from the moment the plane took off until she returned three months later. Immediately on return the pain recurred and at the present time remains unresolved.

Many of the patients seen were involved in long existing life problems which had gradually built up to more or less intolerable situations. It is a condition frequently seen in females in their late twenties; these ladies are generally single and show their frustrations through accumulated tension.

One young lady in her late twenties, fit and athletic developed pain in the left side of her jaw extending to the ear. She was convinced that the pain originated in the lower left molar teeth. X-rays revealed nothing and replacing existing restorations did not alleviate the pain which became chronic. She was finally convinced that her pain was of emotional origin after reading Ruth Moulton's article 'Emotional Factors in Non-Organic Temporomandibular Joint Pain' and once convinced the pain disappeared.

4. **Bruxism**: Whilst the grinding or clenching of teeth may lead to joint problems other sequelae occur. Firstly, excessive wear may occur and this may lead to complete breakdown of the teeth. Secondly, we may see the supporting tissues succumb under the excessive load, the supporting bone and the tissues recede leaving sensitive gingival areas at the necks of the teeth exposed. This process if not arrested is continuous. Thirdly, we may simply get pain following the clenching. Nocturnal clenching is shown when pain is felt in certain teeth which disappears during the day. This pain is due to the stretching of the periodontal membrance, the membrane supporting the teeth to the bone.

Much of the treatment for these conditions has followed a pattern to break the syndrome. For example a denture can be placed in a patient's mouth which will take the teeth out of contact and not allow the satisfaction of grinding. Sleeping tablets or Valium can be given to create a deeper sleep or some relaxation. However all of these things overlook the basic problem, the cause of the habit — the cause of the tension.

Uncontrolled tension is one of the major problems facing the health professions. This recognition being given, our efforts must be away from drugs and placation and toward retraining the mind to a balanced and relaxed situation. This way the intolerant will tolerate, the tense will unwind, we will show better judgement and live happier and healthier lives.

Psychosomatics in Practice

Dr John Walters

THE FACT THAT millions of prescriptions for sleeping tablets are dispensed annually clearly reflects the incidence of insomnia. Yet insomnia is not a disease but a symptom of a more fundamental disturbance in people themselves, in their thinking and in their way of life.

A typical example of a person suffering from insomnia illustrates this problem. Although the individual may be tired throughout the day, on lying down and attempting to fall asleep he finds his body restless and his thinking overactive and stimulated. The body seems to want rest, but the mental activity will not permit spontaneous sleep. Finally after thrashing around for a time he may fall asleep exhausted and wake after a fitful rest feeling tired and washed-out. If this situation is repeated on a number of successive nights the restlessness is aggravated by a fear of not sleeping and the subsequent fatigue. The underlying tension causing this insomnia is primarily a problem of overactive thinking which the individual is unable to control. Because of the large number of thoughts, ideas and memories competing for attention, his mind is continually racing and does not have the capacity to settle or quieten down to a more restful state. With insomnia the physical weariness from lack of sleep is the end result, but the cause lies in distracted and uncontrolled habits of thinking.

The common tricks people use to try to sleep, such as counting sheep, are attempts to engage the mind and settle it. When the mind is quieter the body will not be subjected to such a bombardment of nervous impulses and will relax. In fact, whenever the mind is occupied in some positive activity, the body will be able to rest. For example when we are busy doing some useful task, our mind has no opportunity to think of fears or negative attitudes and we are spontaneously happy and relaxed. It has often been said that the Devil finds work for idle hands and this probably expresses the idea that an undirected mind will be distracted more easily by desires or emotional thoughts.

Insomnia therefore is a symptom of a mind that is uncontrolled or undisciplined. The thoughts of such a mind are not under the individual's control and like a wild animal cannot be trusted until trained to behave consistently. Relaxation can be looked at as the product of a disciplined mind, a mind that has the capacity to concentrate and settle down to its natural, peaceful state.

In seeking to become aware of and control these extraneous thoughts an individual needs to find a practical way of living. In former generations the pace of life was slower and pressures probably fewer; people lived a simpler and more straightforward existence and the problem of tension did not arise as often. In those generations there were other stabilizing influences such as the support of family, a well defined set of cultural and social values and widely accepted religious traditions.

Yet what can be gleaned from this experience of the past that could be fundamental in stabilizing people today? All religious and spiritual traditions advocate the practice of morality, not so much for its own sake, but to enable the mind to free itself of negative distracting thoughts and to attend to more constructive and useful areas of thinking. Nobody welcomes fear, anxiety or worry and yet without a practical philosophy of living, incorporating ethical principles such as patience, honesty or contentment, tension is inevitable.

These principles need to be experienced at a very practical level that directly relates to daily living. If the individual can adopt a calmer and more regulated pattern of living, he may then become slowly aware of negative attitudes within himself that distract and unsettle him. If practised consistently this self-observation must lead to greater discrimination between useful and useless attitudes. If these negative attitudes can be eliminated and their positive counterparts developed, stability and self-awareness must improve. If an individual can practise a little more patience, tolerance, compassion, forgiveness or love, to that extent he will be a more integrated human being.

For the mind to rest after a day of activity it must be stable and quiet, and thus any practice that helps the person relax and settle down will contribute to relieving insomnia. But more than this, such a practice may be the beginning of a life-time of self study and training in living.

It could be said that the totality of this approach lies in a way of life that is moral, a mind that is concentrated and a body that is free to be naturally relaxed. Such a cure is a simple thing to begin, but a far-reaching retraining of the whole person to complete.

* * *

The following case studies further illustrate some

aspects of the management of psychosomatic disease.

Mr. C., a forty-five year old insurance officer, was seen by his general practitioner following a 'turn' at work lasting half an hour. While working he had suddenly collapsed with sweating, shortness of breath, a rapid pulse and breathing, and general weakness. When examined at home he was normal apart from looking anxious and strained. He had recently stopped smoking and had moved down from the country for his work, and these recent adjustments in addition to his general worries, had caused him a lot of stress and anxiety.

Four days after this anxiety reaction he was checked again and found to have blood pressure (B.P.) of 140/100. After having discussed his general anxiety problem he agreed to commence several simple practices. He was given a mental quietening exercise and breathing routine to practise daily.

Several months later he reported that the practices had helped a lot in easing his anxiety symptoms and he no longer had any trouble sleeping. However, because he was generally feeling so well, he had lapsed into inconsistency with the exercises until he finally stopped them.

Mr. C. was not seen for eight months but returned after that interval complaining of a dull chest pain related to exercise. The pain came on after walking 300 yards. His life style had again become pressurized and tense, and he was smoking heavily to 'calm his nerves'. On examination he had B.P. 170/120. Hypertension and myocardial ischaemia (angina) were diagnosed, and he was referred to a cardiologist.

However, within one week he had an attack of severe chest pain at rest, lasting thirty minutes, and was admitted to a coronary care unit of a large hospital and a diagnosis was made of myocardial ischaemia, with probable subendocardial infarction. In hospital he still had a

B.P. of 155/110 and was started on hypotensive therapy Propranalol and Cyclopenthiazide; two weeks later he was discharged from hospital and saw his general practitioner a few days later.

At this visit, still on drugs, his B.P. was normal and he was retaught the mental quietening practice and the breathing routine, which he resumed daily. One month after his discharge from hospital he still had angina after walking a quarter of a mile. From this time he did his exercises regularly each day, gradually incorporating physical Yoga practices as well.

Three months after his hospitalization, he noticed that his exercise tolerance had increased and that the angina was less. Within six months his angina had disappeared and within twelve months his B.P. had returned to normal and he was taking no drugs.

Twelve months after his myocardial infarction, the report of the cardiologist stated that he was: 'Fit and confident with practically no chest pain; B.P. 150/90. Mr. C. has done extremely well and has now virtually no evidence of his previous anterior descending coronary artery thrombosis. It is gratifying that he is free of pain and particularly gratifying that he is free of depression.'

Mr. C. himself ascribed his improvement to the regular practice of Yoga and particularly to his change of attitude. He no longer felt tense at work and was able to fulfil his family responsibilities without worry or anxiety. It was obvious that his whole outlook on life had changed from being fearful, nervous and anxious, to being fit, confident and happy, with a positive approach to his responsibilities and future.

For the ensuing two years he has continued this progress and is very fit and healthy.

* * *

Mr. S., a forty-two year old businessman, relates a long history of hayfever and asthma.

During childhood he suffered from hayfever and skin allergies to grass and pollens through the summer months. In adolescence, respiratory problems developed, including asthma. These became more severe with time.

In his early twenties he developed recurrent bronchitis that was associated with asthma. His doctor blamed the area and state which was believed to be the worst in the world for these complaints. These infections were generally treated with injectable antibiotics, tablets and capsules.

One interesting observation was that he not only had asthma when he went near dry pollen-laden grass but if he looked at a picture of dry grass the effect was the same — a wheezing attack.

At the age of thirty a severe attack of asthma required adrenaline injections and finally hospitalization for two weeks. While in hospital he was treated with oxygen, tranquillizers, antidepressents, antibiotics and broncho-dilator drugs. One week after admission, physiotherapy was commenced and the physiotherapist told Mr. S. that in her experience if he continued the way he was going, he could not expect to live much beyond the age of forty years. The medical staff advised him to learn how to relax but could only offer him tranquillizers.

At this point he took up Yoga and was given breathing practices which made him realize that he could control his breathing rather than the breathing controlling him. There was immediate improvement followed by slow, steady progress as the treatment began to involve him in more than just the physical, mental and breathing practices. The physical well-being that he experienced as a result of the initial practices helped to re-establish his self-confidence and provided the necessary incentive to continue his daily programme of exercises. Within five months his vital capacity had increased from 2400 cc to 4200 cc. He had increased in height and lost excess weight.

Through a process of self-observation he began to learn that self-help was the most important type of therapy and that physical treatment only provides limited relief but does not solve the underlying problem. The problems of fear, lack of confidence and tension required a much more thorough, long-term approach to his total development and integration.

In thirteen years of practising Yoga, he has had no further asthma or allergic problems and has felt progressively more stable and able to contribute to the welfare of others.

Mr. K., a thirty-nine year old businessman, illustrates how by practising Yoga he could stabilize his emotions and thinking, thus benefitting several psychosomatic conditions including thyrotoxicosis.

As a child, Mr. K. went through the normal run of illness and was always very active, highly emotional and impatient. He was often described as a happy person but with this happy mood also came moods of great anger.

As a young man he was physically very fit, competing in athletics, pennant tennis and squash. Up until the age of twenty-six years his resting pulse was 45-55 per minute.

It was at this stage that he noticed he had less energy during sporting events and his resting pulse increased to 75 per minute. Within two years he had a resting pulse of 120 beats per minute, a protruding left eye, a tremor in the hands and extreme emotional agitation. He lost 1¼ stone in weight and developed incapacitating fainting episodes. Thyrotoxicosis was diagnosed by a consultant physician but the condition was not adequately controlled with the drugs prescribed. After twelve months he was recommended to undergo thyroidectomy but feeling unsure about surgery he declined the operation. His symptoms were always worse under pressure and he felt that there was a psychological basis to the condition.

It was in this state that he decided to try Yoga. Having enrolled at a traditional centre, he was given a mental quietening practice and a simple explanation as to the importance of taking decisions and accepting the consequences. Two days after this first session, he was on the telephone taking note of work to be completed when he started to feel faint because of tension in facing such a work load. He sat down, did some breathing, and sat quietly doing the quietening practice. After five minutes he was able to look at the work, decide what was the most important work to do and resign himself to the fact that the rest would not be done. This was done with a clear conscience knowing that he could only do his best; and with this attitude he has avoided fainting for nine years.

In the three months after starting Yoga he gradually tapered off the pills and required no further medication. Over a period of two years his protruding eyes receded and they became stronger with better acuity. More recent thyroid tests have been normal.

In the four years it took to completely overcome the illness he did regular Yoga practices including one posture specifically for his thyroid condition.

An integral part of the cure has been his change in attitude which Mr K. describes thus:

> 'When I feel impatient with a person, I realize I have insufficient tolerance or love and need to try to find something positive or lovable in that person or situation. If I do become impatient I only cause myself mental and physical harm. I feel very fortunate in having this tendency as I am forced to

be vigilant and positive in order to avoid dramatic mental and physical discomfort. I feel the Yoga practices have gradually increased my awareness.'

Psychosomatics in Perspective

The Practitioner

Character in Health

Janet Gudkovs

ONE OF MY FAVOURITE stories is a traditional Indian tale. It concerns Savitri, daughter of a king, who chose a noble but ill-fated man, Satyavan, as her husband. When her choice was made known to the king his advisor, a seer, foretold that Satyavan was doomed to die in twelve months. Because of her love, Savitri stood by her decision to wed Satyavan and went to live with him in the forest. As the twelve months came to an end Savitri spent her nights in fasts and vigils. On the last day she begged permission to accompany her husband deep into the forest where he usually went to cut wood and gather fruit. As the day passed Satyavan was overcome by headache, fatigue and fever, and in a dark part of the forest, died with his head resting in his wife's lap. In the deep gloom Savitri saw a vision of Yama, king of death, come to collect Satyavan's soul and then go on his way. Savitri, faithful to her husband even in death, followed behind. Three times Yama attempted to persuade her to go back, that it was useless to follow, but each time Savitri, convinced that her duty was to be with her husband, answered in such a fashion that Yama could argue no further. Such was her wisdom and devotion that Yama eventually relented and granted Savitri her husband's life.

It seems to me that this ancient story taken from the Indian classic, the Mahabharata, has something to teach the modern psychotherapist or medical practitioner. It suggests that a person with certain qualities, such as patience, courage, devotion to duty, wisdom and love, can heal another who is suffering.

In my understanding there is a factor which relates very fundamentally to the course of human development, to suffering and its alleviation. This factor is character. I am not referring solely to the aspect we describe when we say of a person: 'He has got character', which restricts the meaning of the word to the possession of positive qualities only, or the old-fashioned concept, virtues. Character, in the sense I use the word, is the basis of a person's response to life, whether this basis resides in positive or negative emotions, feelings, impulses or motivations.

In trying to understand man as man, as opposed to man as animal or man as machine, modern psychology focuses on the concept of personality. Thus most humanistically orientated psychologists will espouse one or another theory of personality development, individual differences and personality disorder. However in my view, an understanding of character — its nature, development and pathology — is far more important than the concept of personality in understanding man and his suffering.

Personality is the stamp of psychological individuality in the broadest sense. It relates to the more superficial manifestation and projection of the person. The particular style of thinking and writing, the way a person dresses, his preference in eating, the manner in which he expresses himself — these all bear the mark of his own uniqueness and individuality. Thus, personality accounts for much of the variation in people's nature. Character, however, relates to fundamental principles or absolute values. Thus, the extent to which different people embody such qualities as patience, consistency and responsibility, which are constitutive of strong character, also leads to variation amongst them. However, character and personality are not identical. A person may have a strong personality but a weak character. The personality trait of arrogance, for example, in one person may lead to a disrespect towards others, whereas in another it may be sublimated to self-reliance and the holding of firm convictions. Furthermore, a quality of character such as intolerance may be expressed in different ways because of personality differences. Thus, a quiet person can be just as intolerant or angry as an outgoing boisterous one, but simmer inside rather than express it openly.

To me, character seems to be a factor of more consequence than personality because it is more influential in determining the basic choices a person makes in life and hence the experiences he undergoes and his suffering. A person's response to situations, even when this is not a conscious process, always reflects a choice. Sometimes the response seems to be an automatic reaction; that is, the person does not think about it as it has become habitual. However, that reaction still lies within the ambit of the person's own responsibility because the basis on which the habit has been built rests on the choice they have made in responding to the initial situation.

The point I wish to make here was illustrated in a film which attempted to document the effect of an alcoholic mother on her two daughters. On the one hand, we saw one of the girls responding with embarassment, with resentment and in the end having all the problems in the world, being a disturbed young person and becoming almost antisocial. In contrast, the other girl, even when the mother did wrongly by her, responded in a far more positive way as if to say: 'Look, despite all this, she is still my mother'. There was more forgiveness, more tolerance, more acceptance in this sister at such an early age.

This film helped me understand aspects of my own development and also that of people whom I see during the course of my work teaching and counselling. While there are often various upsetting situations and problems in a person's background, somehow it does not seem to help to blame the environment saying: 'I am like this because such-and-such happened to me'. The way in which a person has responded to that environment seems to be decisive in whether he or she is left with resentment, with guilt, depression, anxiety and so on. If an individual's own desires or fears have been uppermost, emotional reactions with their consequent tension are inevitable. For example, simple observation will show that a person who is impatient, who cannot wait, who wants his own desires satisfied immediately, will always be tense. If there are many situations to which he reacts impatiently, tension becomes chronic and the subsequent diversion of energy from organic and other vital functions of the body may eventually precipitate a psychosomatic condition. The crucial point is whether his response has been based on a narrow, selfish interest or on a more altruistic one. This choice is fundamental to human existence. A person can choose what is convenient, what is easy and involves least effort, what satisfies his desires, or he can choose to respond in a more detached, altruistic fashion which releases him, creates self-respect, integrity, peace and stability.

At each point in time these decisions register within the person; that is, there is always a part of the mind which knows whether an action has been selfish at the root level or unselfish. If someone chooses to ignore his conscience, its sensitivity diminishes, although I believe that the registering, at a deeper level, does not cease. In this context it is also important to understand that a person has a history, a memory and hence an accumulated register of decisions or choices. I have observed that if one consistently decides to do something selfish rather than something unselfish, it registers in a fashion that creates the feeling 'I am not good; I am bad'. This in itself is a form of suffering or stress and can ultimately release a self-destructive mechanism within. This is one way in which physical symptoms may be precipitated in the body. Another way they may be precipitated is through the need for attention. A person who is lacking self-respect, who has no love for himself, is constantly seeking the reassurance of others and may invent a disease condition in order to achieve this.

It is necessary therefore for a therapist or doctor to look at his or her patient's whole life pattern when treating a disease condition, for it is not just the current situation or stress that should be taken into account, but the person's habits of thinking, feeling and acting which have cumulatively added up to his present suffering. An awareness of the energy equivalents of thought processes makes the type of thinking a person allows himself to entertain very important. To discover those thoughts and attitudes which release energy and sustain the vitality of the body-mind complex is a subjective study incumbent upon anyone who is attempting to heal others. Knowing the means by which a person may come to achieve a greater control over his thoughts and feelings, and an ability to sublimate those which are negative and hence have a detrimental effect on his health and happiness, is vital if a therapist is going to be able to effect a lasting change for the better in his patients.

Humanity in Medicine

Kenneth Ingbritsen

AT THE PRESENT TIME there is considerable discussion about the effectiveness of our technological and drug-oriented practice of medicine in combating the seemingly ever-increasing incidence of psychosomatic disorders. Many people are succumbing to the pressure, stresses and strains of a materialistic society built on competition and emphasizing worldly success. Consequently, fear of failure creates much anxiety and tension for the individual who is constantly competing with his fellows for wealth, status, power and other symbols which signify that he is better than the next man. Therefore, the medical practitioner is continually confronted with the results of this approach to life, whether they be physical, emotional or mental in character. In these cases prescription can only remove the symptom, not the cause of an individual's disease or illness.

Therefore, we must ask the question: in what way can a medical practitioner become more effective in relieving the suffering of his fellow human beings? The skills he has assimilated and practised in medical school are no doubt useful tools, indeed extremely important in his practice of medicine. However, of greater importance are his qualities as a person, whether he can practise medicine and use its tools humanely. Unfortunately, the growing reliance on science and technology to solve man's ills has led to the neglect of personal resources and knowledge that could be developed in the treatment of disease. Perhaps the fear of failure, so common in all areas of our community today, and the inability to come to terms with suffering, have caused us to negate and even deny our innate ability to understand and comprehend an individual's problem to the point that the only knowledge we consider worth trusting is mechanical and technical.

In seeking to answer how a medical practitioner becomes more effective, we must determine the knowledge he requires for correct diagnosis and treatment. Perhaps this could be related to the following quotation from an ancient Ayurvedic physician:

> 'The science of life shall never attain finality. Therefore, humility and relentless industry should characterize your every endeavour and your approach to knowledge...The entire world consists of teachers for the wise and enemies for the fools. Therefore, knowledge conducive to health...coming even from an unfamiliar source should be received, assimilated and utilized with earnestness...'(1)

These words, written 3000 years ago by Punarvasu Atreya, seem as relevant in the twentieth century as they were then. To expand on this Ayurvedic concept, there is nothing that can be experienced or conceived that does not influence the body or the mind of the individual to a lesser or greater degree. Since anything that affects the constitution one way or another can be utilized as a therapeutic agent, there is nothing that is not medicine. This idea is perhaps at variance with our Western concept of medicine as practised today. However, it does place emphasis on a total approach to health in which all phenomena should be considered: physical or physiological, psychic or emotional. This approach also differs from the conventional one in that it does not try to prescribe treatment en masse, but considers each individual as shaped by heredity, environment, character traits and many other factors. This approach demands more of the practitioner in terms of his knowledge of man.

This knowledge of man has to be of a very practical kind. We see our schools and universities preoccupied with research and the validation of theories. Yet is this the type of knowledge conducive to reducing human suffering? The following stories should clarify this point.

The first story concerns a professor, who in his travels came to a ford which had been flooded. Concerned that he had an appointment to keep, he asked assistance of a villager, who kindly arranged for a boat to take him across to the other side. As this villager ferried the professor across the river, the latter asked of the villager: 'Have you ever studied philosophy?' The villager replied that he had not. Contemptuously, the professor exclaimed: 'Then you have wasted half of your life!' Just at that time the boat sprang a leak. The villager turned to the professor and enquired: 'Have you ever learnt to swim?' The professor replied very tersely that he had not. The villager commented: 'In that case you have wasted the whole of your life.'

The second story involves three clergymen, each from different faiths, who attended a conference together. One afternoon they had no session to attend, and so decided to try their hand at fishing in the nearby harbour. They hired a boat and made their way to what was considered the best spot for fishing, and cast their lines. After several hours one of them realized he had promised to ring his wife and so apologized to his two fellow fishermen, and made his way to shore by walking on the water. Not long after, the second clergyman excused himself also, and made his way to shore in the same manner as the first. Now the remaining clergyman was quite dumbfounded by all this. He pondered to himself: 'My faith is no less than theirs, surely I can do the same.' Then he stepped over the side of the boat, and went straight to the bottom. He struggled back on to the boat, and not convinced that his faith was any less, tried again, with the same result. Just then the two clergymen who had previously excused themselves made their way along the shore, and witnessed what was happening. As the third priest went under for the third time, one of them turned to the other and remarked: 'Do you think we should tell him where the reef is?' Quite often the knowledge we receive through our education is only theoretical and does not help in coping with many of life's situations, irrespective of vocation.

In general terms, the current education system provides the technical and skill development for an individual to take his place in the community as related to his career or job. Yet, especially when we talk in terms of bringing into our professional or personal lives the quality of humaneness, we find the present system of education sadly lacking. Perhaps this is better stated if it is put in the form of a question: What type of knowledge does one need to become a humane person? Most would agree that it is desirable for the practice of medicine to be humane. In fact, we could go so far as to say that if the humane element in the practice of medicine is missing, then there can be no effective cure, especially of psychosomatic disorders.

The qualities of a humane person are compassion, a deep inner conviction and dedication to serving the needs of those with problems, consistency, a sense of responsibility, patience, honesty, integrity and confidence in his own knowledge, and in the case of a doctor in his capacity to heal. The present system of education is not really equipped to provide this training.

And yet, can a patient trust, and have confidence in, any practitioner who does not exhibit most of these qualities? To a certain extent progress can be made where a patient believes in the drugs, or the technical gadgets used by the practitioner. However, underlying all effective treatment is the capacity of the practitioner to understand the individual on all levels — physical, mental, emotional and spiritual. If the practitioner is ignorant of any one of these aspects, how can he bring to bear on a particular problem all the required knowledge to make an accurate diagnosis and provide treatment which will attack the cause or root of a problem rather than alleviate the symptom?

This deep insight and understanding of human nature begins first and foremost with the practitioner's understanding of himself — his motives, his fears, inhibitions and potentials. How many practitioners have seriously thought about, or are aware of, their motive for involvement in the practice of medicine. Is it the financial rewards which attract, or the status, or power? Maybe they are fulfilling family expectations, or perhaps they are genuinely motivated to serve their fellow man as medical practitioners. The nature of the motive will determine their effectiveness as healers.

If motivated by financial reward, status, power or other such factors, the practitioner's ability to care for his patient is limited by his selfishness. If this is the case, the practice of medicine is purely a means to an end, and to that extent the patient, as a human being, is of little importance to the practitioner. He is to be used as a ticket to a dollar, to a bigger and better home, to a position of authority and status. With the practitioner's concern being gain and not the patient's problem, lip service only is paid to ethics. The patient will not relate to a codified system of ethics printed and bound sitting on the practitioner's bookshelf. He will relate to the doctor, to his approach, and assess whether his example is of a person genuinely motivated and concerned to meet his need for help. If he does not find that in the practitioner, no matter what is prescribed, the patient cannot be expected to have full confidence in the treatment.

However, if the practitioner is motivated to understand his fellow man's needs, and provide him with answers he so desperately wants, he should pursue with 'humility and relentless industry' the knowledge required to make himself an effective healer. This would inevitably mean that he would need to make an assessment of his capacities, both at a professional and personal level. Let us put aside professional capacities for the moment, and consider what other personal capacities are required for a medical practitioner to be effective. The practitioner must search himself to understand what capactity he has to love. All the previously mentioned attributes of a humane person are components of this quality. All too often we see in our community that most people want and expect love, but are unwilling to give it. Very rarely do we come across a person who has developed this capacity to love his fellow human beings to the extent that he is consistently benevolent, compassionate, tolerant and understanding. Very rare in our community is the man who will sacrifice his own personal needs for those of another. And yet, particularly in the field of medicine, love is the cornerstone without which there can be no humanity; there can be no real individual or social progress towards a sane social order and/or identity as a peaceful, happy community.

If one is sceptical of this purported power of love, then in our own jargon people like Pitirim Sorokin have provided an explanation which is scientifically sound. In his book, 'The Ways and Power of Love', he explains how an understanding of natural principles of living can be discovered, assimilated and experienced by those who go beyond the logical, the technical and the intellectual to an inner, more spiritual source of knowledge.

We see in our present-day community the results of a lack of love. From a lack of love there is a deep-seated insecurity, whether it be in the child who has missed out in receiving parental love; or in the husband or wife disenchanted with their relationship because they find the other unlovable; or whether because of the competitiveness, greed and desire for material possessions, love for one's fellow man is put aside and exploitation replaces a genuine care and concern. The resulting anger, frustration, resentment, alienation and suffering manifests itself socially in the phenomena of physical and mental breakdowns and disease, apathy, excessive emotionalism, drug abuse and misuse, violence and suicide.

It is from this background and in this social context that the practitioner's patients are drawn. It can be simply stated that what all the patients who seek help require is genuine care, attention and reassurance that as individuals they are worth caring for, for it is through the care that they re-establish a respect for themselves. If a practitioner assesses his capacity to love, he must first become aware of the factors which actually prevent him from loving. These factors are his own needs, desires, inhibitions and those subconscious tendencies conditioned in time by various factors such as family upbringing, education, peer group relationships and the environment. This awareness of the forces and inherent tendencies which guide his behaviour and determine his capacity to cope with the demands and stresses of living in an affluent, materialistic society, is the first step in the gradual release of his potential to love.

Therefore a person who can heal is that person whose psyche is free from fears, inhibitions and negative tendencies which normally prevent him from relating to the total patient in a humane way. A person whose psyche is overwhelmed by selfish thoughts and preoccupied with fulfilling his or her own needs cannot possibly empathize with or give his full concentration to the needs of the patient.

More often than not, instead of making an effort to increase his capacity to love he takes the easy way out — believing that through the use of science and technology he can actually help the patient. This by the way is not an attitude peculiar to medical practice only; it has permeated the whole fabric of our society. What is really happening is that the practitioner is ashamed to face a person who is suffering, knowing he does not have the capacity to fully comprehend that person's problems and provide any answers. In fact he has not integrated the various facets of his own personality and character to the extent he can consider himself sufficiently emotionally stable and well-adjusted to cope with any pressures or demands made on him. Consequently the relationship with the patient is depersonalized. The practitioner puts that patient at arm's length by subjecting him to a confusing and bewildering barrage of tests after which he is in no position to question the practitioner's ability to heal.

How often do we see a professional flounder in his personal relationships, for example, in his family life, as a parent or as a neighbour, even though he is very adept in his professional life. This lack of training in being able to relate, not only to a patient, but even to one's own social group at more than a superficial level reflects a lack of guidance and principles of living from which to develop a framework to understand one's own experience. Consequently, adhering to a system of professional or medical ethics without living life in an ethical manner is tantamount to promoting the hypocrisy which is already rife in all sectors of community life.

It is time medical practitioners took a deeper look at themselves. Perhaps with consistent training and the development of self-awareness they will find a store of intuitive knowledge far more powerful and infinitely more effective than the tools, gadgets and technology in which they currently put their faith.

The development of this type of knowledge requires an ongoing commitment to one's personal growth and self-development. And it can be said with reasonable surety, that, as few people ever become perfect, there is always room for improvement and refinement in ourselves as human, indeed humane beings.

1. 'Yoga Pracharak' Vol 9/No 2, Yoga Education Centre, Melbourne (1973)

Reflections of a Bystander

Dr John Funder

As MOST OF MY professional life has been spent as a pathologist in a metropolitan hospital, my association or involvement with patients has been largely indirect. However, for some years now I have taken a special interest in psychological medicine. My interest stems from having attended lectures and discussions related to psychosomatic disease and from attentive listening to the modes of treatment proposed for the somatic and psychological components of the disease in question. I have read a modest amount of contemporary writing regarding clinical psychology and psychiatry. On occasions I have sought counsel from a number of people including clinical psychologists and psychiatrists and have been asked by friends to recommend counsellors for themselves, their relatives or their friends.

Inevitably, such an interest takes one into broader fields, such as sociology and philosophy. And I find it very heartening that barriers between the great cultures, philosophies and religions of the world are being broken down. As one who has been moulded largely by the traditional Judaeo-Christian culture of the West, it has been a very enlightening experience for me to learn of some of the great richness of Eastern religious and philosophical systems. This has come about largely from my personal encounter with the Director and staff of the

Yoga Education Centre. I find quite credible the statement of the historian, Arnold Toynbee, that historians of the future may well consider the most decisive cultural development of the twentieth century the beginnings of dialogue between the great religions of the East and of the West — more decisive than the tragic wars of this century or the confrontation between capitalism and communism. Such considerations are certainly relevant to a consideration of psychosomatic disease. For however much new and improved technologies may contribute to the understanding and management of psychic disorders, it is surely true that a deeper understanding of the human mind and spirit, culled from centuries of tradition in all of the great philosophical and religious systems of history, will be of great value in the prevention and management of psychic components of disease. To reject such an accumulated wealth of understanding is surely blindness and arrogance.

In the management of the psychic component of psychosomatic disease, the two main types of treatment, apart from that directed to the somatic component, are presumably drugs and counselling. Here, my interest lies only in the counselling side of the psychotherapy.

There seems to be a considerable and growing number of theories or schools of thought regarding modes and types of counselling. Perhaps the large number of theories is itself an indication of the somewhat primitive state of the sciences of psychology and psychiatry.

However, I find one very encouraging sign in this confusion. It is admitted that success in counselling is dependent to a very significant degree on the character of the therapist. A number of psychiatrists will have different success rates, using the same techniques of counselling. And a number of psychiatrists may have a high success rate, using different counselling techniques.

For me, this shifts the attention from the mode of therapy to the therapist.

Reflecting on my own experience and that of my friends, and on my reading, I have tried to examine the personal qualities of three counsellors whom I have known and whom I regard as competent and effective. Do they have a common quality or attribute, 'a highest common factor', which may be the determinant in their ability to help other people by their counsel?

Here I come to an imponderable — literally an imponderable, incapable of being weighed or measured. For the common quality of the three people I have in mind is that each one impresses me as a man of deep and genuine spirituality. Of its nature spirituality is imponderable, as it relates not to matter, but to the spirit of man. For me the spirit of man is no less a reality than the matter of which the body (the soma) is composed. For me the spirit is not part of, or a mere expression of Shakespeare's 'mortal coil' which each of us will 'shuffle off'. Discussions on this subject with my medical colleagues rarely prove decisive. We come away from them 'unconvinced', I retaining my stance, as described above, the other retaining his stance that our total being is 'just a matter of chemistry'.

To come back to my three counsellors, what they have in common is not related to a common 'religion' or 'meaning system'. One is an agnostic humanist, one is a yogi and one is a Christian. Each has settled for his own 'meaning system', in the framework of which he has developed his spirituality. Each seems to have achieved within himself a peace and serenity and seems to be 'in control' of himself and of his relationships with his fellow men. In these relationships each shows the qualities of love, caring and compassion, and a firm ongoing commitment to the service of his fellow man.

Words such as 'caring' and 'compassion' recur in the literature of psychotherapy, but too often it seems to be assumed that they are qualities which we naturally possess and have no difficulty in practising consistently. This is certainly not true. These deeply human and humane qualities must surely be acquired by a painful process of growth within ourselves.

If there is validity in what I have written, it seems essential to incorporate and stress the process of self-development in the training of clinical psychologists and psychiatrists. As far as I know little, if any, emphasis is placed on these considerations in contemporary training curricula — but I am subject to correction in this matter.

Practical difficulties certainly exist, but the benefits arising from such training would certainly greatly outweigh difficulties which would have to be overcome. The process of spiritual growth, of a greater degree of self-realization, would certainly demand periods of withdrawal and periods of silence. Such periods of withdrawal and silence would conflict with contemporary training curricula, which appear to be highly competitive and crammed with requirements related mainly to knowledge of techniques in psychotherapy.

Some part of what I have written is reflected in the closing section of Viktor Frankl's 'Man's Search for Meaning: An Introduction to Logotherapy'. Under the heading 'Psychiatry Rehumanized' he writes: 'For too long a time, for half a century in fact, psychiatry tried to interpret the human mind merely as a mechanism, and consequently the therapy of disease merely as a technique. I believe this dream has been dreamt out. What now begins to loom on the horizon are not the sketches of a psychological medicine, but those of a humanized psychiatry. . . . Our generation is realistic, for we have come to know man as he really is. After all, man is that being who has invented the gas chambers of Auschwitz; however, he is also that being who has entered those gas chambers upright with the Lord's Prayer or the Shema Yisrael on his lips.'

There is a final point. For each of us, whether or not a trainee in psychology or psychiatry, the path towards spiritual growth and self-realization is not only difficult but is beset with pitfalls and dead-end sidetracks. A guide and teacher is needed for a safe, forward journey. And the question arises: 'Who shall be our guides and teachers?'

Part Two

Psychosomatic Medicine: Eastern and Western Approaches

Is Yoga Healing or Therapy?

Shri Yogendra

THE DIFFERENCE between art and science is axiomatic, because while art is creative and therefore flexible, science is invariably precise. In curing diseases — physical, mental or otherwise — success is sometimes achieved through art and sometimes through science. In treatment, art is associated with healing, prayer, meditation etc., while science identifies it with therapy like surgery, Ayurveda, Unani, Allopathy etc.

What is Yoga in relation to the treatment of disease — is it healing or therapy? Yoga is a total process both of healing and therapy for all ailments in life.

Instances are not wanting about persons having been cured of many supposedly incurable diseases through Yoga both in the past and the present. These are often referred to with reverence and pass as miracles. Drugless systems like naturopathy are now using Yoga practices and this admixture has given a new slant to the prevailing confusion. With such confused perspectives, it is becoming difficult to evaluate Yoga either as an art of healing or as a therapy.

The cures effected by Yoga have been variously ascribed to both healing and therapy. Healing is generally associated with the art of curing a disease with spiritual or faith cure achieved in some inexplicable form. Yoga healing in this sense — often passing as miracles — is a form of theotherapy which recently has been fully recognized as a permissible method of treatment in the wards of nine hospital groups in London. The word healing is a misnomer in the strictest term since the process is governed by a subtler law of cause and effect which must have a scientific base not sufficiently known to us. In fact, this approach to the treatment of disease has much in common with the art of healing through psychosomatics. Yoga healing through an obscure instrumentality undertakes the restoration to a normal condition — the medical term being homeostasis.

Therapy implies the application of remedies in the treatment of disease. This may fall under various categories, i.e. with the aid of internal medicine, surgery or otherwise. Yoga as therapy has a store of methods which although primarily preventive and hygienic have also the merit of therapeutic utility. Because the total application of a cure depends, in the case of Yoga, both on healing and therapy, we have preferred to term the integrated process as yoga psychosomatics. Although uninvestigated Yoga maintains a scientific approach to the problems of disease and its treatment.

From the medical works of the ancient Indians, it is known that both the yogins and the students of Ayurveda had recourse to the dissection of dead bodies to gain full knowledge of anatomy and physiology. That certain information on the working of the human body was available to the yogins is evident from many older Yoga texts. Besides, there are also records of the Chinese and other travellers which detail many remarkable cures of chronic diseases yielding to yoga psychosomatics. Institutionalization was a common feature and the patients had to stay at the hermitages of the various yogins. Even texts on applied Yoga dealing with physiology and biology have dealt with the treatment of various diseases through a certain combination of Yoga practices, for example: respiratory, gastric and nervous disorders through the combination of various forms of physical therapy, zone therapy, hydrotherapy, intermixed with mental and spiritual therapies better understood now as psychoanalysis, psychiatry etc.

In Yoga, diseases are conceived as being three-fold: saririka or biologic, manasika or mental, and adhyatmika or psychic. That a disease is an interrelated syndrome is hardly understood or appreciated by modern science to the extent it should be, although psychotherapy, psychiatry and similar methods have been recognized as science. That, in fact, there are no qualified physicians who could treat any disease in its threefold aspects except the yogins is known.

Consequently, each aspect is treated independently by the practitioners of their respective systems without regard to the interrelated influences of other parts of the whole. For example, apart from mental abnormalities, psychic diseases were given no credit as having any baneful influence upon the general health of an individual. Yoga has emphasized for ages that no diagnosis or curative system is complete or really successful unless and until it also includes investigations in and elimination of the cause-potentials affecting the various planes of life.

This ancient wisdom of the yogins is now anonymously being recognized by many open-minded and progressive research students of medicine and psychotherapy. For instance, the unitarian doctrine of disease as a disorder of personality — body, mind and spirit — emphasized by the ancient yogins has only recently been scrutinized and enriched in Italy by the eminent physician and surgeon, Nicola Pende — the Founder of the contemporary school of medicine called Neo-Hypocratic. According to this new doctrine, hormonal and humoral disturbances and maladjustments give rise to constitutional and correlative antagonisms, whether chemical, nervous or psychic. What is produced is a disease — in fact, a disorder of the Whole Man and thus of the body — owing to an impairment of the vital response of the body itself. 'In the normal state of health, this response regulates all the different parts of the body and is put into effect through the humoral system. On this account, man is always a totality and an individual (sui generi), and disease is always a disease (totius substantie)', no matter whether the effects are felt by the body, the mind or the spirit.

Yoga does not base its treatment on chemical, herbal or any extraneous measures, nor does it believe in treating the symptoms of the disease but their cause. Rousseau merely repeated, as it were, the old yoga truism that 'Hygiene is the only part of medicine, and hygiene is more a virtue than a science'. In Yoga, the emphasis has always been on the merits of hygiene, preventive and social medical education or discipline, purificatory and constitutional autoprocesses of regeneration of the tissue cells, regalvanizing of metabolism and other similar measures.

It is admitted that statistical data in favour of yoga therapy was wanting because the average yogin was concerned more with curing the sick than in maintaining records of his achievement. For the first time in the history of yoga therapy, however, case records and statistical data have been kept and analyzed from 1918 onwards by the pioneer institute of scientific Yoga, The Yoga Institute. What is more impressive is the case of illustrations of refractory — chronic functional — diseases which yield to no other medical measure as they so successfully do through yoga therapy. It is logical therefore that instead of a priori prejudice against Yoga, the subject is given the same opportunity which other systems of medicine enjoy so that the best may be proved in the interest of suffering humanity.

Psychosomatic Diseases in Ayurveda

Pandit Shiv Sharma

AN AMERICAN FRIEND once asked Mahatma Gandhi why his disciple, J.C. Kumarappa, used violent language when denouncing the British Rule in India, while he himself meticulously avoided the use of such language. The Mahatma replied that, in assessing the violence of J.C. Kumarappa's anger and the sharpness of expression, provision should be made for his Madras diet which was full of chillies and hot spices.

On the face of it, it is a lighthearted remark, but that great man never treated any question lightly. This reference to the effect of diet on an individual's nature and behaviour involving both body and mind, was based on his observation of, and belief in, the phenomenon which had been noticed, studied and described in detail in the earliest Ayurvedic texts.

Man, according to Ayurveda, is a somatic-cum-psychic-cum-spiritual being. The food he eats, the water he drinks, the air he breathes and the physical, mental and spiritual activities he pursues, are all interrelated and interdependent. There is nothing about man that is exclusively psychic or exclusively somatic. Everything is psychosomatic.

Ayurveda takes an extremist stand on this issue. A boil on the skin is a local phenomenon, so is a minor bruise anywhere on the body; but it soon becomes a psychosomatic phenomenon in the case of a neurotic and offers his mind a base for displaying various neurotic attitudes. Conversely, mere mental stress can result in a boil or even a crop of boils and their continual recurrence which disappears as soon as the mind is free from stress.

The concept of man as a psychosomatic being was introduced in Ayurveda later during its development. The system began with the concept of tridosha as the fundamental principle on which the entire edifice of Ayurveda has been built. Under the tridoshic concept it is impossible to divide the human being into two independent entities, the physical and the mental.

The word 'tridosha' means 'three doshas' — vayu, pitta and kapha. 'Dosha' has been translated by some scholars as 'humour'. This school of translators has equated the doshas of Ayurveda with the 'humours' of Hippocrates. However, it will not be possible, within the scope of this small paper, to dwell at length on the reasons why the doshas cannot be interpreted as humours, but the Ayurvedic profession, as a whole, has rejected this translation as misleading and incorrect. The Ayurvedic doshas are the three irreducible basic classifiable metabolic psychosomatic constituents, or, rather, constituent-complexes of living matter. Unlike humours, the doshas pervade the vegetable protoplasmic matter as much as the animal protoplasmic matter. In other words, the tridoshic concept is biological and covers all animate matter.

Ayurveda has divided the human being into three psychosomatic types, the vata-prakriti, pitta-prakriti, and kapha-prakriti. Just as there is some analogy — though no real identity — in the case of the Greek humours and Ayurvedic doshas, there are many similarities between the abovementioned three dosha-prakritis, and Dr W.H. Sheldon's three basic types, ectomorphs, mesomorphs and endomorphs as described in his work 'The Varieties of Human Physique'. Here it becomes necessary to introduce the Ayurvedic definition of medicine: 'Nothing exists in the world (of thought or experience) that is not medicine'. Since the term medicine covers every thought, word, action, experience or substance that exists in the world, there is nothing we can think of or perceive through our senses that is not medicine.

The kingdom of man is an aggregate of the three protoplasmic function-complexes of vayu, pitta and kapha, which maintain the smooth flow of healthy life when they are acting in harmony and balance. Disharmony and imbalance constitute disease. The role of medicine is to restore the harmony and balance. Therefore, a factor, in order to be called medicine, has to influence the doshic balance in varying degrees and directions. In this sense, whatever affects the stability of the body chemistry is medicine.

Everything that exists falls into one or more of the three categories of the vatic, paittic and kaphaic factors. Thus the sun is paittic and the shade is kaphaic or vata-kaphaic in nature. A stimulant is a paittic drug and a sedative a kaphaic drug. An alcoholic drink, being paittic, will increase the paittic activity in the body and the anti-paittic or kaphaic coconut water will counter the action. Again, anger will promote the paittic activity in the body, cheerfulness the kaphaic and the antipaittic activities.

Matter, in order to be animate, has to be tridoshic. Life is inconceivable in the absence of even one of the doshas. An ideal balance between the activities and the structure of the three respective doshic factors constitutes the normality of the constitution from the metabolic viewpoint. However, absolute normality is a myth as the constitution from the metabolic structure fluctuates not merely from individual to individual but within the individual himself. It is the predominance of the activity of a particular dosha in an individual that decides his type and not the total absence of the other doshas. Even where a dosha is predominant, the activities of the non-predominant doshas cannot fall below a certain minimum level in the living protoplasm. If the imbalance exceeds the limit of the latitudes within which the minimum tridoshic equilibrium must be maintained to make life possible, the organism ceases to live. Between this lowest limit and the absolute normal there exist innumerable combinations and permutations of the tridoshic activities which represent as many deviations from the normal.

It has already been stated that the doshas are not the humours of Hippocrates. A dosha is more a synergistic hormonal psycho-physical activity-complex than a humour. The tridoshic complex, therefore, should be translated in English as physico-physio-psychological organismal phenomena-complex.

From the above it becomes clear that in the very basic Ayurvedic concept of the constitution of the human being there is no room for isolation of the physical from the psychic phenomena or vice versa.

The doshic manifestations themselves are twofold, normal and non-normal, or healthy and unhealthy. Enthusiasm and fear, courage and anger, steadiness and laziness, exemplify the respective healthy and unhealthy manifestations of the three doshas, vata, pitta and kapha, on the psychic plane. Similarly, physical agility and lightness of limbs on the one hand, and pains, stiffness and aches in the body on the other, are both vatic characteristics on the physical plane. The former is the manifestation of the vata dosha in a healthy state, the latter manifests the vitiation of the vata dosha. The degree of vitiation, both at the somatic and psychic levels, is determined by the degree of 'deviation from the normal' (vikriti) and the severity of the resulting symptoms. The aim of the treatment is to correct the deviation and restore and maintain normality.

At the psychic plane, a single emotion may be di-doshic; e.g., cheerfulness is a kaphaic emotion but if it turns into intense joy, the happiness is kaphaic and the keenness or the thrill of it vatic. In steady courage, courage is basically paittic but the attribute of steadiness is kaphaic, and if the emotion partakes of the attribute of enthusiasm which is vatic, the emotion becomes tri-doshic.

Despite the fundamental inseparability of psychic and physical disease in Ayurveda, there has to be some sort of division for practical handling of the patients.

Although the Ayurvedic physician is not to lose sight of the psyche while treating what appears to be an exclusively (that is predominantly) physical disease; and similarly, not to ignore the body while dealing with the psychic illness, the separation of the two categories has been achieved successfully to such an extent as to lead to bifurcation of even epidemics into physical and mental and even moral varieties. As an extreme example we can take the statement of Punarvasu (600 B.C., or earlier) that immoral or improper behaviour also leads to epidemics.

In the same vein the vitiated psychology of human beings is described in Charaka Samhita, an ancient Ayurvedic text, as a real factor in psychic epidemics:

> 'When the leaders of a country, city, town or village take to immoral behaviour in their dealings with the public, then the dependents and subordinates surrounding them aggravate the immorality. The

immoral behaviour eclipses the duty, honesty and religion and that land becomes godforsaken.' (Charaka, Vimana III, 24-25).

Immorality, asserts Ayurveda, cannot be conducive to the peace and happiness of the community and vitiates even the normalcy of the elements of nature, the qualities of the soil and produce, and even the seasonal phenomena like rainfall, heat and cold. It is not necessary, however, for a materialist to accept this view; but the general ethical approach to world problems which follows as a necessary corollary should be accepted by everyone. As the Charaka Vimana says: 'As the age of truth declines, some people find themselves in possession of too much adana. This leads to heaviness in body and lethargy in mind, which leads to fatigue, which in turn results in laziness, then hoarding and taking what belongs to others, and greed and avarice. This chain of demoralization goes on through treachery, falsehood, uncurbed desire, anger and wrath, vanity, hatred, cruelty, shock, fear, distress, sorrow and anxiety. Then the bodies and minds of the people deteriorate and become ready prey for disease. Thus even the span of life is lowered.'

The treatment of mental disease in Ayurveda consists mainly of awakening the mind to higher values through meditation, realization of truth, bringing back into the conscious mind suppressed memories, etc.

It may be helpful to emphasize the difference between the psyche and the brain. This difference has been well brought out by an experiment conducted by three eminent Indian doctors of the Physiology Department of the All India Institute of Medical Science, New Delhi. The experiment consisted of keeping the hands of some yogis in ice-cold water and studying the monopolar EEG scalp recording before and during deep meditation. The EEG recording started showing blocking of the alpha rhythm before the subjects going into deep meditation, after two or three minutes immersion of the hand in cold water at four degrees Celcius. This was a natural reaction as would occur in any other case. But once the yogi entered deep meditation, his right hand remained immersed in ice cold water for as much as fifty-five minutes and no discomfort or pain was felt by him as was demonstrated by the alpha activity in the EEG record, which remained undisturbed throughout the entire period of immersion. The EEG record is a strictly physical phenomenon as it records the electrical activity of the grey matter, and not the thought processes of the yogi. The structure of the nerve cell in the brain in the normal condition, existing before the yogi goes into deep meditation, cannot be physically changed. The only change that can occur, and which the yogi can bring about by detaching his thoughts completely from the external world around him, can be in his own mind. Whatever may be the aim of the experimenters in conducting this study, the results of the study unmistakably proved that the yogi utilized his mind to retain the normality of the alpha rhythm in the EEG record, which the normal individual could not do under identical circumstances according to current scientific thinking.

This paper has laid comparatively greater emphasis on the psychic aspects, as the modern scholar or medical scientist is generally less conversant with its place in Ayurvedic literature.

At his clinic, the Ayurvedic physician has to carefully take stock of all psychic as well as the somatic factors governing the conditions which bring the patient to the clinic. In this set-up the heredity, the race, the family, the culture, the psychology, the environmental influences, the social, dietetic, educational, geographical, climatic and constitutional factors, including those of age, disease-resistance, general tone, physical strength and individual idiosyncrasies, are all carefully considered. The physician has to establish a rapport with the patient. Sympathy and solicitude, in the psychic cases in particular, go a long way in gaining the confidence of the patient. This is supported or supplemented with the use of drugs, diets and practices. The last three cover a very vast area. The importance of the study of these three categories assumes great significance in view of the Ayurvedic belief that you cannot standardize the treatment by merely standardizing the medicines. The inability of any science, ancient or modern, to standardize the patient, means that the standardization of treatment can be termed so only when it is subordinated and adjusted to fit the total psychosomatic personality of the patient. Therefore, the study of the constitution of the patient, in all its fluctuations, is very important in marshalling the aid of the three categories to the best advantage of the mind and body of the patient.

People have lived on hopes and died on vitamins. No single factor by itself can suffice for dealing with the total man. When all the three categories are utilized, keeping in mind the physico-physio-psychological factors involved in the 'illness' of the patient, the treatment assumes a truly psychosomatic approach towards the establishment of the normality of the total man.

Psychosomatic Aspects of Traditional Chinese Medicine

Dr Yasuo Otsuka

ONE OF THE MOST popular Japanese proverbs says, 'Yamai wa ki kara', which means that all diseases come from ki. Ki (ch'i in Chinese) is an important concept in Chinese natural philosophy and also in medicine. Ki is therefore very often used in the daily conversation of Japanese people, who adopted this notion from the Chinese as early as the 5th or 6th century. Byo-ki (disease) is literally the suffering of ki. 'Ki o ushinau' (one loses ki) means that one loses consciousness. 'Ki o otosu' (one lets one's ki fall) means that one is disappointed. 'Ki ga kuruu' (one's ki comes out of order) means that one becomes mad. 'Ki ga wakai' (one's ki is young) means that one is mentally young for one's actual age. From the above examples we see that ki is something which makes a human being alive and human-like. A man without ki is nothing but a cadaver. But ki can function only in the presence of karada (human body). The first example of ki, 'yamai wa ki kara', means in the sense of the contemporary Japanese that all diseases occur or can be aggravated through psychic movements. From another point of view ki is breath or air. Ko-ki (inspiring of ki) is inspiration. In the ancient Confucian literature on the rites of the state Chou (ca. 1100 B.C. — 256 B.C.) the following interesting remark is given in reference to the confirmation of a man's death: 'Let a piece of cotton come near to the nose of a patient and confirm that ki ceases to move.' Ki is therefore on the one hand air as a natural phenomenon and on the other hand something which plays an essential role in physiological and mental activities of the human being. Similiar concepts from other ancient cultural areas, are psyche or pneuma in the Greek and prana or atman in the Indian.

According to the Chinese tradition ki circulates with ketsu (hsieh in Chinese and phenomenally blood) in the human body and makes every part of it work in order. If the circulation of ki or ketsu is disturbed, a disease may occur. As for ki or ketsu the former is ranked higher than the latter. Ketsu is made from ingested foods or, in traditional expression, five sorts of taste and in its turn supplies every part of the body with necessary nutrition to maintain the morphological basis of each. Even ketsu is for itself an inanimate substance and becomes animate only through activation by ki.

To sum up, the human body consists of different sorts of organs, which for themselves are isolated inanimate entities. Through the activation of ki they become animate and work with each other in close co-operation suiting the purpose of the living organism. Ki is therefore the highest agent to control the somatic and the psychic activities of the human being. In this respect the somatic and psychic activities are inseparably connected with each other in Chinese medicine.

In Chinese medicine emotions are considered not to be seated in the brain but dispersedly in various organs. According to the go-gyo (wu-hsin in Chinese, five evolutionary phases) theory, anger is seated in the liver (wood), pleasure in the heart (fire), thinking in the spleen (earth), grief in the lungs (metal) and fear in the kidneys (water). But each of them does not operate independently, having influences on the others, facilitative or inhibitive. As for the facilitative direction, the liver acts on the heart, the heart on the spleen, the spleen on the lungs, the lungs on the kidneys and the kidneys on the liver, while as for the inhibitive direction, the liver acts on the spleen, the spleen acts on the kidneys, the kidneys on the heart, the heart on the lungs and the lungs on the liver. An example: excessive anger causes hyperfunction of the liver, which in turn depresses the function of the spleen. Another example: the hyperfunction of the kidneys causes the hyperfunction of the heart and excessive pleasure.

This principle was used also in medical practice. Chang Ts'ung-cheng, one of our four greatest physicians in the Chin and Yuan-dynasty, was famous for his psychosomatic treatment. In his work 'Ju men shih ch'in' some case reports are given in which psychosomatic thoughts are fully employed. One of them is as follows:

> 'A woman of a rich family had been sick with troublesome thinking and sleeplessness for two years, and medicinal treatment appeared not to be effective. Her husband asked Dr Chang for treatment. Dr Chang examined the patient and said, 'The pulse of both wrists is soft, which indicates that she is suffering from a disease of the spleen, because the spleen is the seat of thinking.' Chang asked the husband how he could anger her. Then for several days continuously the husband spent lots of money on drinking. The patient flamed with anger and fell into a heavy sweating and exhaustion. She collapsed into a deep sleep. After that she was freed from sleeplessness and loss of appetite. The pulse recovered as well.'

This example is an application of the above given logic 'Anger depresses thinking.'

Nowadays the relationship between physicians and patients has become unfortunately all the more estranged. Physicians are more interested in laboratory findings than in the patients' complaints. Even if patients are suffering seriously, physicians can give them nothing but tranquillizers, providing they have no special laboratory findings. The patients are of course not satisfied. Tranquillizers are in short non-specific depressants of the central nervous system. In this process no attention is paid to treating a patient as a specific individual. In traditional medicine non-specific central depressants are not used. For a patient with sleeplessness the medicine used should be effective for the particular patient but not effective for sleeplessness in general. Physicians used to say, 'This medicine is not a hypnoticum. Therefore it may be that you would not sleep fifteen or twenty minutes after taking it. If you want such an effect, you can get medicines for such a purpose from any doctor. Your sleeplessness is a product of both your psychic and somatic illnesses. This medicine will improve your condition and as a result of course your insomnia will be cured.'

One of the major reasons for the revival of traditional medicine in Japan lies in the fact that traditional medicine takes more interest in human relations than Western medicine. From ancient times the importance of human relations between physicians and patients has been repeatedly stressed in this medical system.

The following episode of Kuo Yu, a famous Chinese physician in the first century, shows the importance of human relationships in treatment:

> "A noble once asked Kuo Yu for treatment. Kuo Yu failed to cure him, although he was one of the best physicians of his time. The emperor, wondering why, let the noble clothe himself as a poor man and

sent him again to Kuo Yu. How marvellous! The patient was cured by one needle puncture. The emperor asked Kuo Yu for the explanation. Kuo Yu said: 'Medicine is will. . . the nature of the skin is so fine that the slightest failure could provoke an unexpected result. Physicians should employ the greatest caution in the ki-circulation of patients. Success depends on the state of the heart and the hands of the physician. The 'How' is something to be realized and never to be explained. 'However, nobles behave, in general, haughtily. So, I engage in my work with a sort of fear. Furthermore there are difficulties in the treatment of nobles as nobles assert a will of their own and do not trust me.' "

Traditional medicine is a system in which diagnosis and therapy cannot be separated. In other words, in the traditional system patients are classified according to therapeutic means, while in the Western system diseases are classified according to pathologic findings. In the former a patient is diagnosed as one who is to be treated with the formula so-and-so, and in the latter as one with gastritis. And what is more, it is said that in the traditional system every diagnostic procedure has at the same time a therapeutic meaning, positively or negatively. A glance, a word and every possible act of a physician have influences on a patient, and are sometimes even more important than the so-called therapy. If a physician seems to be lost in thought and puts his head on one side, a sensitive patient could guess that he might be seriously ill, which could aggravate his illness.

As already mentioned, ki is considered the highest agent for keeping physiological and mental activities of the human being in order. When the ki-circulation goes out of order, a disease may occur. In order to recover the disturbance of the ki-circulation we use various sorts of treatment; physical, dietetic, medicinal and others, of course on a psychosomatic basis. Acupuncture is one of the most important ways of healing in the Chinese tradition. We know fourteen cardinal meridians and some other supplementary ones on which a series of treatment points are located. The meridians were originally considered as passages of ki. Acupuncture might have been devised as a modification of blood-letting, a widely used technique in the ancient world. After the formation of the concept of ki, people came to think that if a needle puncture could influence the ki-circulation, blood-letting might not be necessary. Today nobody doubts the effectiveness of acupuncture against certain diseases.

Medicinal treatment is the core of traditional Chinese medicine. Jo-ki, one of the most important directions of this treatment, means to bring ki into normal circulation. Gonzan Goto (1659-1733), a famous Japanese physician presented the theory 'ikki ryutai setsu' (all diseases are the result of the disturbance of the ki-circulation). The most prevalent theory of pathogenesis in his time was the theory 'san in setsu' (theory of three causes). According to this theory there are endogenous, exogenous and non-endogenous-non-exogenous factors responsible for the occurrence of diseases. The excess of seven sorts of emotion: pleasure, anger, grief, thinking, sorrow, fear and astonishment belong to the endogenous factors. Six climatic conditions: wind, coldness, hotness, wetness, dryness and glow belong to the exogenous factors. The intemperate life such as diet failure or sexual indulgence belong to the non-endogenous-non-exogenous factors. Goto said: 'These three factors could cause disease. But unless the ki-circulation is disturbed, no disease occurs. Under the same coldness some become sick and others not.' Because of this point of view he very often used so-called ki regulating preparations along with balneotherapy, bathing in a waterfall and moxibustion.

The revival of traditional medicine is an international phenomenon. This phenomenon seems to be paradoxical, because it occurs at the moment when Western medicine is growing with incredible speed. But the more technical progress is made, the less humanistic thought is taken into account. Western-orientated physicians are interested in traditional medicine chiefly because of the expectation of unknown pharmacologically active substances. If such substances have been discovered, they want to use them in the context of Western medicine. This is of course a possible approach to enrich the medicinal therapeutics. But patients may expect other things in traditional medicine. Newly developed substances supplement Western medicine, but do not complement it. Traditional medicine should be used and developed in a context of its own. The psychosomatic nature of this medical system could work only in this way and thus it could complement the Western system of medicine.

Yoga Psychology

Dr C.T. Kenghe

YOGA HAS BEEN a very important feature of Indian culture from time immemorial. The Vedic seers were great yogins and even in the age of the Indus Valley Civilization, yogins were highly respected. Yet throughout the ages, Yoga has remained shrouded in mystery for common people and even today in spite of wide proliferation of Yoga, real Yoga continues to be a treasure of very few practitioners. The advanced yogic techniques were considered to be too secret, of course not without sufficient reason, as even today humanity cannot be said to be ripe enough to use these techniques properly. Yet, if human civilization is to be saved, man will have to return to Yoga proper and make himself fit to practise real Yoga. Most of the Yoga centres and institutes today are propagating only pseudo Yoga, concerning themselves with a few physical exercises for health and cheap techniques for meditation not necessarily sanctioned by the tradition. Very few even try to understand real Yoga, let alone practise it. Hence a sincere attempt towards understanding Yoga should be looked upon as a welcome gesture.

Although what is usually called psychology today can hardly be said to be the concern of Yoga, psychology in its original and literal sense is certainly the subject-matter of Yoga. Today, psychology has become mostly a study of behaviour and behaviour is studied by conducting experiments on animals and animal aspects of man. Yoga on the contrary tries to enter into the farthest depths of human personality and to actualize the highest potentialities of mind by removing the impurities that come in the way of such an actualization. Again, unlike traditional psychology based on Greek philosophy, Yoga is an exact science and not a speculative system. It is the most practical study and not an abstract theory regarding mind and its behaviour. It is for this reason that this science can be most useful even in the context of modern life. Let us now examine the findings of Yoga in respect to mind and its nature and the methods it has evolved for tackling the mind.

Although we are all aware of our minds, it is by no means an easy task to define the mind. Several working definitions were tried by Western psychologists and now the quest has been almost abandoned as hopeless. Yoga has a very definite idea of mind. It defines mind as the power of cognition as distinct from pure consciousness in itself which is said to be the nature of the soul. The brain may be said to be the organ which manifests and utilizes this power with the help of the central nervous system, but the power itself cannot be identified with the brain, just as the electric powerhouse can be said to be the mechanism that manifests and utilizes the power of electricity, but the power itself cannot be identified with the powerhouse, That eternal power functions through different brains Brains may be born and die, but the power is eternal, deathless. To stretch the same illustration further, electricity is eternal although the generators and powerhouses are certainly destructible. Thus mind is neither brain nor its effect, but the eternal power that works through the organisms of the brain.

For understanding the exact nature of mind, it should be properly differentiated from soul; especially because there has been a lot of confusion in this respect among Western thinkers. In Yoga, mind is not looked upon as the source of consciousness. It derives consciousness from another source viz. soul. Thus it is not self-conscious or self-luminous. Patanjali (author of the Yoga Sutras) states clearly that mind is not self-luminous in so far as it too can be made an object of consciousness. We are aware even of our minds and thoughts and to know this is most essential for tackling mind. Postulation of another mind cannot solve the problem as it would lead to argument ad infinitum. Thus, according to Yoga, mind also is an object. Actually it becomes not only the medium of knowing external objects, but the whole of the objective universe is evolved out of mind only. It is thus the very source of the objective world.

Four stages of natural evolution have been recognized by Yoga. The first is the original unevolved state having no distinct mark of its own. Yet it contains three primordial forces called sattva or the force of light and purity, rajas or the force of energy and activity and tamas or the force of inertia and darkness. These forces are in the state of equilibrium or perfect balance and so none can become more prominent than others. When equilibrium gets disturbed due to contact with subjective reality or pure consciousness in itself, the second stage arises in which the sattva becomes more prominent due to reflection of consciousness within it. This stage can be called pure or universal Mind. This mind further evolves to form the sense organs and subtle matter which is the third stage. It is in the fourth and final stage that the subtle matter gets further evolved into the gross matter. Thus matter comes at the rag-end of evolution according to Yoga and the Original Nature or the evolving principle can in no way be called material. It may be called mental, for mind is the very first outcome of natural evolution.

Patanjali calls mind citta which literally means 'that which is made conscious', indicating clearly that it is not self-conscious or the source of consciousness. Besides this word, Patanjali has occasionally used the words manas and buddhi to denote certain particular aspects of mind. Manas denotes the volitional and emotional aspects whereas buddhi denotes the rational and cognitive aspects of mind. Citta covers all these aspects. It is the main instrument of the spirit or subjective reality both for enjoyment as also for self-realization and liberation. For the sake of enjoyment, it evolves into different types of organisms and perceives the objective world as also the sense organs. For perceiving the external objects, mind is aided by the senses. According to Yoga, mind is a changing and transforming principle. It is said to go out actually through the senses and to assume the form of the respective object. It is thus that the object becomes known. But the mental modifications themselves are known by the spirit who is said to be immutable. The spirit does not assume the form of mental modifications, but just illumines them with consciousness. It is hence that the mental modifications are always known whereas an external object may be known or may remain unknown. It is known when mind assumes its form in its epistemological process going out through the necessary sense organ, but when it does not transform itself in this manner, the external object may remain unknown.

In Yoga, the general functioning of mind is usually compared with that of a river. Through waves and ripples, the river comes into contact with the external objects, but the dirt and mud collected through such contact also give their colour to the waves. Similarly mind comes into contact with external objects through its modifications and then the further modifications get the colour of the experience arising out of such a contact. Mind in a pure state is needed for the self-realization of the spirit but the mental modifications coloured with impurities blur the image of the spirit. This happens due to the forces of rajas and tamas implicit within the Original Nature itself. For gaining self-realization, the first and foremost requirement is to make the mind pure by removing the impurities. However, the impurities can be removed only by diving deep into the mind, and for entering the depths first of all the surface is required to be made steady. This surface mind consists of the constantly flowing modifications. Hence Patanjali defines 'Yoga as the inhibition of the mental modifications'. It may well be remembered that modifications in themselves are not harmful, but the impurities which give their colour to modifications make them so. When the impurities are removed, a steady flow of clean modifications reveals nothing but liberation of the spirit in its real nature. Hence, modifications are to be inhibited only as a prerequisite for removing impurities.

Patanjali has classified mental modifications on the principle of cognition for the convenience of study, although in themselves the modifications are extremely varied and innumerable. Thus, for the sake of study these modifications may be brought under five headings which can well be shown to be exhaustive. Applying the principle of cognition we can easily see that the modifications may represent the objects, emotions and thoughts as they are, or it may be an erroneous presentation of any of them, or it may concern just verbal ideas having no perceptual correspondence in reality, or it may be just an absence of objects, emotions and thoughts, and lastly the modifications may be concerned with some previous experience of any of the five types lingering in the mind. Beyond these varieties called valid knowledge, false knowledge, ideation, deep sleep and recollection respectively, no other type of cognition can be imagined. Yoga is not concerned much with the study of these varieties for themselves and hence they need not be discussed here in detail. The real concern of Yoga is with the impurities or tensions with which these modifications are usually infected and of which they can well be freed by applying certain techniques.

Although in Western psychology the concept of the unconscious aspect of mind is considered to be the discovery of Sigmund Freud, Yoga has given a much more consistent and definite theory of the unconscious long, long back. It has described in very clear terms the mechanism responsible for the formulation of the unconscious. This mechanism consists of four tensions, all of which function on different levels of consciousness and repress the memory traces and impressions of actions and experiences to form what may be called the personal unconscious. These four tensions are (1) 'I'-persona or self-assertion, (2) likes or attachment, (3) dislikes or repulsion and (4) clinging to life or fear of death. These tensions are the impurities which prevent the light of consciousness from reaching the depths of mind just as the muddy water prevents the light of the sun from reaching the depths of the river. When any one of these tensions becomes quite prominent, it suppresses the others and becomes obvious by rising to the surface mind in the form of a modification. But this is not usually the case. Usually more than one tension remains equally prominent and thus due to conflict the flow of tensions gets intercepted. The flow of tensions is also intercepted owing to the control of the moral sense or what Freud calls the 'super-ego'. In such an intercepted condition of tension a person may even simultaneously love and hate the same object or the same person and it may culminate in serious disorders of personality. It is mostly under such an intercepted condition of tension that the various mental complexes are formed. For freeing ourselves from the trouble of these complexes, first of all, we are required to bring all the conflicting tensions to an attenuated condition for which Yoga has prescribed some useful techniques. However, for removing finally the basic cause of the troubles, we are required to get rid of these tensions and of course of the mental modifications infected by them. Some tensions remain completely latent awaiting a suitable opportunity to make their existence felt. However, even these influence behaviour adversely. Hence, during the course of the yogic practice, a practitioner is required to tackle even such tensions by bringing them to the conscious level. These tensions have been defined by Patanjali in very clear terms. However, they cannot be discussed within the short span of this article.

Yoga has a very clear-cut theory as regards the contents and working of the unconscious as well. It should be remembered here that it remains unconscious only till it is reclaimed by applying the yogic techniques. Having known these techniques, Yoga can speak of the unconscious in clear terms whereas Freud and other modern psychologists are very vague in this respect. Thus seven properties of mind have been described in Yoga as those that are not fully seen and these can well be said to be the contents of the unconscious. These are — (1) inhibitions, (2) latencies of moral and immoral actions, (3) subliminal impressions, (4) mutations, (5) vitality, (6) activity and (7) potentiality. First of all, there are inhibitions, formed by repressions. Several of our instincts do not get proper scope for expression due to social fear etc., and get repressed. These have been discussed at length by Freud and other modern psychologists. Yoga, however, goes beyond repressions. According to it, all our past deeds, though forgotten as far as the surface mind is concerned, remain as latent drives in the unconscious and influence behaviour. These deeds may have been done during this life or during the previous lives of the person concerned. Their latencies remain firmly attached to the person and actually direct the whole course even of his conscious life. Thus the unconscious has its roots in the prenatal period and mind cannot be said to be the tabla rasa even at the time of birth. This can be said to be the special feature of the Yoga view of the unconscious. The unconscious is carried through several lives and through its unseen force determines the next type of birth, the span of life for the same, as also enjoyments and sufferings to be experienced in that life. The functioning of this unseen force is based on the mechanism of tensions. Moreover, Yoga firmly maintains that the unconscious is not a mere storehouse of repressed memory traces, but carries beneath them a great potentiality for attaining psychic and spiritual powers and prescribes definite techniques which any sincere person, through practice, can utilize.

Besides this concept of the personal unconscious, Yoga has also conceived of the collective unconscious in the form of the fifth tension called nescience. This nescience always remains completely latent or at the deepest unconscious level and provides the field for other tensions to grow. This is common to all persons in so far as it consists of initial error of not perceiving the difference between subjective reality and objective reality and thus becomes responsible for evolution in mind generally. We are all born with nescience and all our experiences are based upon nescience although for practical purposes we differentiate valid knowledge from false. It is this nescience that makes us see permanent what is impermanent, pure what is impure, pleasure what is pain and self what is non-self. Through advanced practices of Yoga, even the collective unconscious can well be tackled and ultimately even the initial error can be corrected.

For entering the depths and reclaiming the unconscious, Yoga has prescribed inhibition of the mental modifications as the first requirement. For bringing the most unsteady surface mind under control, continuous practice is required along with the attitude of dispassion. The subtle psychological process that happens while entering the depths is called the conscious Yoga. It consists of four stages. In the first stage, we try to arrest our customary images so stopping the activity of the conscious mind, the complexes in the unconscious get gradually resolved and the repressed drives start rising up in the conscious mind in the form of memory. These usually consist of violence etc. and disturb our mental balance. However there is no need to worry. If these are mentally followed with a deep understanding that they can result only in endless suffering and ignorance, we can easily get rid of them. This is called the technique of contrary suggestion. As long as these drives remain repressed, they cannot be removed. But once they rise to the conscious level, a firm contrary suggestion is sufficient to get rid of them. After this trouble is stopped, meditation continues quietly for some period and then the trouble again arises as the further depths are reached and subtle complexes are resolved. In the second stage, we are required to follow the subtle drives and get rid of them with a similar technique of contrary suggestion. Then in the third stage, the practitioner starts experiencing a deep state of rapture or ecstasy in which he feels the supreme joy or delight. However, that is not the goal. It is only the sign of re-absorption of the tension of clinging to life into the tension of repulsion and then that of the tension of attachment.

For overcoming this tension also, the practitioner is advised to follow up this joy itself and thus transcend it. Then this tension also gets re-absorbed into the tension of self-assertion. In the fourth and final stage, the practitioner is advised to follow up and get rid of this tension and so reclaim the whole of the personal unconscious.During the last two stages of the conscious Yoga, the practitioner already starts experiencing psychic powers. Yet the goal is not reached as the basic tension of nescience, forming the collective unconscious, remains to be transcended. This is to be achieved by remaining unattached to the higher faculty of knowledge by means of the supreme attitude of dispassion.

Mental modifications can also be inhibited in another way. This can be done by catching hold of the gap in the flux of ideas and then trying to extend it as much as possible. Thus a complete void or the notion of stopping all mental experiences can be reached. This is specially recommended by the Buddhists. The mental activity can also be stopped by means of the physiological manipulations prescribed in Hatha Yoga for suspending all physiological activities. Thus temporarily all mental modifications can be inhibited. However, the unconscious remains untackled and forces the practitioner to return to the same type of objective experience once again, sooner or later. Hence, to tackle the unconscious the Buddhists have prescribed five things to be practised along with this path. They consist of (1) openness of mind without any prejudice and predilections, (2) special vigour and energy, (3) recollection, (4) contemplation and (5) intuition of the faculty of higher knowledge. Through these means also the personal unconscious can be reclaimed and the collective unconscious then transcended with the supreme attitude of dispassion.

Thus, Patanjali has not given any place to God and religion while defining and explaining Yoga. Yet, he recognizes the psychological significance of God and religion in reaching the goal of Yoga quickly and without hindrances. Even then he does not accept God as the creator of the universe or helper of devotees in any way. The practitioners can derive only some psychological advantage through the concept of God as a special personality untouched by tensions, fruition of actions and passions. By repeatedly bringing such a concept to a mind as also by repeating the monosyllabic word 'Om' expressive of God, a practitioner can realize the nature of the Self as the inner-most pure consciousness. Not God-realization, but self-realization is considered to be the goal of Yoga. Even traditional religion can help in this respect by bringing the tensions to the attenuated condition. It is worthwhile to note that belief in God and religion is by no means a 'must' for Yoga and that Patanjali has left the option open in this respect and prescribed other techniques for those who cannot have any firm and unswerving faith in God.

Patanjali has described nine aberrations of mind which hinder progress in the path of Yoga. These mental aberrations are (1) ill-health, (2) boredom, (3) doubt, (4) negligence, (5) laziness, (6) incapacity to withdraw from objects, (7) delusions and hallucinations, (8) not reaching the required stage of progress in the yogic practice, and (9) inability to remain there even after reaching the same. These can well be called psychosomatic disorders and neurotic conditions and their concomitants have been described in Yoga almost in the same manner as in modern psychiatry. These are (1) physical pain, (2) distress and depression, (3) nervous disorders,

(4) disturbed inhalation, and (5) disturbed exhalation. Patanjali has prescribed a number of remedies for correcting these disorders. These include interpretation of dreams and free association with relaxation, which have been recommended by modern psychiatrists as well. However, there are many other techniques which also can prove useful in modern psychiatry. The most important remedy suggested by Patanjali is meditation in whatever way one may be able to practise it.

As a general course of practice that can suit most of the practitioners, Patanjali has recommended the Yoga of eight aspects consisting of (i) abstentions, (ii) observations, (iii) postures, (iv) bioenergy control, (v) withdrawal of the senses, (vi) concentration, (vii) meditation and (viii) contemplation of the absolute. The first two aspects are guidelines directed towards cultivation of character. They consist of a code of social conduct and a code of personal conduct. As natural instincts and drives are required to be controlled through these practices, there is always a danger of opposite impulses disturbing the mental balance and Patanjali has prescribed a technique of contrary suggestion as an antidote to the same. The code of social conduct consists of the five virtues viz. (i) non-violence, (ii) truthfulness, (iii) non-theft, (iv) continence, and (v) non-accumulation. The code of personal conduct includes (i) purity, (ii) contentment, (iii) fortitude, (iv) self-study, and (v) surrender to the will of the absolute. Patanjali has given the norms indicative of perfection in these practices which cannot of course be easily reached. It is only after considerably advancing in the practice of all the aspects of Yoga that one may expect to reach these norms.

The next three aspects of the main eight-fold discipline have been called the outer aspects by Patanjali. They are (i) bioenergy control, (ii) posture, and (iii) withdrawal of the senses. They are outer in relation to the three subsequent aspects in so far as they involve some physical effort on the part of the practitioner. However, Patanjali has stressed their deep psychological significance. The posture has been defined as that which brings in stability and happiness. This can collectively indicate the various meditational postures as also the corrective ones. In the practice of postures, Patanjali has particularly advised avoidance of unnecessary effort and to try to merge oneself in the infinity. Such a practice results in the non-clash between the pairs of opposites. The postures have deep neurophysiological significance and if properly practised they can restore neurophysiological balance by removing the tremors. Bioenergy control (prana) is to be practised by regulating respiration. However, bioenergy should never be identified with breath. It is a subtle vital energy forming a sheath between the physical sheath and the mental sheath. It can thus affect both mind and body. Patanjali defines bioenergy control as the interception in the movement of the in-going breath and the out-going breath, after the posture is mastered, four varieties of bioenergy control have been described as (i) that in which the outer function is controlled, (ii) that in which the inner function is controlled, (iii) that in which the stable function is controlled, and (iv) that which transcends all, having no consideration of the inner and outer functions. These conditions are to be achieved respectively by mastering exhalation, inhalation, retention and sudden retention without complete exhalation or inhalation. Until the fourth variety is reached, the three functions are required to be watched in respect of space, time and number. When watched in this way, the respiration becomes prolonged and subtle. When one gets full control over the bioenergy by regulating respiration, the veil over the force of light gets attenuated and the mind becomes fit for different types of concentration. The last of the outer aspects consists in withdrawing the senses from the sense-objects. This is to be achieved by cutting off contact between the senses and their respective objects and then making the senses imitate the nature of the mind. With such a practice, full mastery over the senses can be well established.

The last three aspects of the main eight-fold discipline have been called the inner aspects in relation to the previous aspects. However, in relation to the seedless state, these too are said to be the outer aspects. The three aspects are concentration, meditation and contemplation. In concentration, the mind is to be tied down to a particular region inside or outside of the body. Retaining the same type of ideas continuously flowing is called meditation. The same meditation is said to culminate into contemplation when it is as though it loses it nature and only the object remains shining forth. These three practices when put together are called constraint (samyama). After long practice the mind passes through three successive stages instantaneously and thus they can be said to have come together. Such constraint releases the potentialities of the mind stage by stage. Seven successive stages in the growth of such a higher faculty of knowledge have been described by Patanjali.

In recent times, some scientists have turned their attention towards the study of the paranormal powers of the mind. Several instances of telepathy, clairvoyance, psychokinesis, precognition etc. have been noted. However, the scientists have not been able to find out how and why these phenomena occur. Hence, the new science of parapsychology is not getting general recognition from scientists. Yoga may prove to be of much help in this respect. According to the Yoga theory of evolution, mind is the source of matter and not vice versa. Hence by understanding the nature and functioning of mind, the whole material universe can be brought under full control. This is the most important theory of Yoga, which modern parapsychology must try to investigate if it wants to get a scientific status. If mind is really proven to be beyond Nature and its laws, it would be extremely difficult to build up a systematic science of the same.

The powers of mind as described by Patanjali appear to be fantastic and infinite. Modern researchers in parapsychology have been able to record only a few. This may be due to the paucity of advanced subjects. Most yogins are reluctant to be subjects for scientific investigations and experimentation. They have been advised not to indulge in these powers and especially not to demonstrate them because attachment to these powers may distract the practitioners from the final goal of Yoga. It would not, however, be proper to consider on this account that the powers described by Patanjali are only imaginary.

Although Patanjali has mentioned that these powers can be inborn in some persons and that they can be gained through some psychedelic medicines, incantations, penance etc. as well, yet the real and important means of getting these powers actualized is samadhi or contemplation. How in the practice of contemplation, different powers are released stage by stage has been explained in detail by Patanjali. Instead of trying to find persons with powers like this, if modern investigators try to train suitable subjects in Patanjali's way of contemplation and go on noting the results, most probably they will be better rewarded and parapsychology will progress faster.

The final goal of life for which the practice of Yoga is prescribed, is to make the personality completely free from all complexes and to get all potentialities of the mind actualized without remaining attached to them in any way. In such a state of mind, termed self-realization, the image of the spirit or soul does not get blurred and shines forth in its real nature. A realized person alone crosses beyond the transmigratory existence and is not forced to be reborn into the world of objective experience.

Yoga Versus Psychology

Dr Robert Sherman

WHAT I WILL ATTEMPT here is a preliminary comparison between Yoga and Western psychology so that you can perhaps understand what our experience is like.

A good place to start is the nature of reality. The West holds that material existence is real. The universe and all its manifestations are real. We can come to know reality through our senses and/or rational process. But our senses present a problem. There is much disagreement as to whether sensation and perception are objective or subjective processes. There are many theories on both sides. But the important point here is that for the Western therapist there is nothing higher than the material world, at least that is as far or as much as he can deal with in therapy. The individual therapist may have some conceptions of 'God' or 'something higher' but these are not part of the therapeutic process. With this view we can come to know reality through our senses. Whenever there is a disagreement as to a particular 'fact' of reality, it is left up to a kind of vote with the majority ruling. This process is termed consensual validation.

Yoga also believes matter is real. But alongside matter is spirit as an ultimate constituent of the universe. Yoga says that the material universe is real but impermanent, as it is the nature of matter to be constantly changing. Spirit on the other hand is permanent and unchanging. Spirit functions as pure consciousness. It is omnipresent but totally inactive. There are two very significant conceptions here. One is the idea of matter as real but impermanent. From it stems the rejection of all materialism. Yoga says that one cannot derive permanent happiness or satisfaction from something impermanent (matter). The conception of spirit as pure consciousness is also highly significant. After some early philosophical attempts to define consciousness, Western thought, especially psychology, has given up the attempt.

The behaviourists openly state that as consciousness cannot be measured it does not exist. The psychoanalysts talk about conscious and unconscious processes but they cannot tell you what consciousness is either. They have a vague idea that as certain phenomena occur in the body there also occur some mental phenomena. It is not necessarily felt that one causes the other but they both happen at the same time. This is called psychophysical parallelism. I do not think it would serve any purpose to go into this any further here, but not only does Yoga talk about what consciousness is, it also outlines a number of distinct levels of awareness that are dependent upon the level of development of the individual. Suffice it to say that in every individual there is a separate spirit. All spirits are equal in terms of qualities and capacities.

So our first major difference lies in the conception of reality. The West stops at the material plane while Yoga goes 'beyond' to a level of spirit. This is the fundamental difference that will generate everything else that I will have to say. The most important result of this difference is the ultimate goal of each process. Psychology must stay within the bounds of material reality while Yoga transcends this reality for something higher.

At this point it might be worthwhile to talk about the nature of man and purpose of life. We in the West have a great deal of difficulty with the purpose of life and where and how we 'fit in'. This seems to me to be an outgrowth of our materialism. We measure the meaning of life in terms of accomplishments, possessions, power, etc. We literally measure and grade all our experience, be it physical, mental or emotional. Even those of us with some altruistic inclinations are concerned about our 'contributions' to others.

Western psychology has this same approach. It views man as a biological organism (sometimes mechanism). It seeks to understand man in terms of measurable traits. All our psychology is based on the assumption of normative behaviour. But far more important is how this gets translated into life. The ultimate for Western psychology is adaptation or adjustment. The healthy personality is one that is comfortable in its environment. This is the manifestation of materialism in psychology and this has led to some serious repercussions. Everything that is considered 'natural' or 'desirable' in man results from this materialism. One example is our notion of aggression. To be aggressive in our society is considered a positive trait as long as one is a male and he expresses this aggression in socially acceptable ways. The therapist actually encourages such behaviour. In fact he considers such behaviour as instinctual and necessary. Now because he takes this position, the therapist must also come up with a theory as to why this aggressive instinct is not natural for females and therefore when one encounters an aggressive female she must necessarily be maladjusted. But I am getting away from my original intention. Western psychology seeks to maintain man as a part of his world. Much criticism has been levelled at therapy as a process of trying to adjust man to a sick society. I do not think it is necessary for me to go into this. The therapist views man as functioning on the basis of id, ego, and superego. The id is the source of primary drives such as sex, aggression, hunger, survival and death(?). The superego is our conscience. The ego is the mediator between the two. The ego is our reality tester. The therapist strives to strengthen our ego — the stronger the ego, the 'healthier' the individual. The psychoanalytic theory of mental illness states that as a result of previous experience we become fixated at a given point in our development. For the neurotic and psychotic, life is a process of trying to satisfy the needs that are generated by this fixation. The therapist tries to make the patient intellectually and emotionally aware of his fixations. Once this insight occurs it is felt that the patient will be in a position to live his life based on his present wants rather than past needs. In a nutshell, this is the goal of therapy. Health is the ability to live in the present. By this is meant the ability to relate to a given situation based solely upon the stimuli at hand. I believe that I am here stating the goal of therapy as best and as favourably as I can. This is (was) my goal for therapy — both as a patient and as a therapist. This goal is really a beautiful thing and very few people ever attain this end. But this again is a very limited materialistic conception of experience within the Western framework, because the yogi also tries for this type of experience. For the yogi this experience means something different and is only the beginning. For the sake of brevity I shall call this experience the quality of 'being here now'.

'Being here now' is in the West limited to sensory experiences. This was (is) the basis of sensitivity training, encounter groups, Gestalt therapy, Rolfing, and many others. These techniques concentrate on developing the awareness of what is going on within oneself at the moment it is happening. Most of us are not aware of what is going on within ourselves. These techniques also emphasized the translating of 'being here now' to relating to other individuals. This leads to greater honesty and perhaps greater 'depth' in the relationship. All of these are very positive qualities and are to be desired by all so long as they do not lead to greater attachments within the relationship. Yoga would point to the limitations of this approach. One manifestation of the limitation of these techniques was that as they grew in popularity in the 1960's and 1970's, these group experiences soon turned into a socially acceptable way to act out one's sexual needs and fantasies. In fact, the group leaders often encouraged this behaviour by emphasizing sex within the group. Now in the West this was both good and bad. But this is not my point here. Yoga would point to this and say, when the ultimate reality is the world of the senses then the ultimate experience cannot transcend the senses. This, I believe, is an extremely important point that I cannot emphasize enough. Since the therapist's view is limited by his materialism the best his patient can hope for is to achieve the same limited view.

The Western man seeks mastery of his environment. With increased control it is felt that increased health, success, prestige, etc. also come. All this, it is believed, stems from an integrated ego. So in summary, Western psychology seeks to achieve a state of psychological health, which is based upon knowledge (insight) of one's motivations, desires, limitations, needs, etc. Control is the key word here because psychology and especially psychoanalysis views man as being basically evil. This is a slight overstatement but the point is, that it is felt that man's basic nature must be either repressed or sublimated. Now sublimation is an interesting concept. It is considered to be the height of enlightened activity. Sublimation is the rechanneling of sexual impulses into creative behaviour. Again, the worth of the individual is measured in terms of his production and contribution to society. Now in one sense this is not so bad for it is perhaps only through sublimation that society is possible. The point that I am trying to emphasize is that even with sublimation the criterion is materialistic. The value of one's 'self' is always measured along a materialistic continuum. Yoga also looks to sublimation as a means of achieving. In the yogic process one controls one's sexual impulses not for the purpose of creation or material gain. In Yoga, sublimation is part of the process in which the spiritual seeker gains control over his entire being so that he can attain a state of extreme introspection without any disturbance. No power of creation is sought or desired as a result of this process.

Yoga has no problem with the purpose of life. The yogi believes that the entire universe, all of matter, is in a constant state of evolution. It is therefore the purpose of life to try to develop or evolve one's awareness to the highest state possible. Yoga believes that it is possible for an individual to achieve the ultimate within his life. But what is this ultimate? Yoga says that the ultimate must be something which is permanent and unchanging. This ultimate is called pure consciousness (or awareness).

Each individual has within him a spirit. This spirit has unfortunately become involved or identified with matter. This can manifest itself with the conception that 'I am my body'. But more importantly, it manifests itself in the form of an ego which separates a particular individual from his experience. The ego falsely identifies itself as the source or awareness or power of knowing. This is a difficult concept to understand. Yoga says that the power of knowing (consciousness) lies only within the spirit within us. Everything else, our mind and body, is only unconscious matter. The mind is separate from the spirit and possesses no awareness of its own. But it seems to us to possess awareness and because of this arises the feeling of ego. Yoga says that this is a form of false perception or ignorance.

It must be understood that Yoga does not deny the existence of ego. Quite the contrary, it states that ego is a part of the basic structure of one's mind (Yoga really does not use the word mind — it talks about the personality complex which includes our concept of mind). Yoga says that the ego is a structural defect of the mind. Just for your information there are five such defects: ignorance, ego, attachment, aversion, and love of life. Yoga says that it is possible to overcome these structural defects through the techniques of Yoga. Once these defects are overcome, or at least brought under control, it is then possible to attain higher levels of consciousness than are ordinarily available to us. The ultimate state is one in which our spirit is no longer bound or involved with matter (our personality complex) and we in effect become pure consciousness directly.

Now I have already outlined some glaring differences between psychology and Yoga. The first is the nature of reality. Psychology believes in the material universe as the ultimate. Yoga says that while matter is real it is impermanent. Yoga therefore concentrates on spirit as its ultimate. Psychology strives for a strong, integrated ego as the means for attaining the ultimate. Yoga says that the ego is both a source and manifestation of ignorance and is a hindrance towards real growth. In Yoga the ego must be overcome. Psychology measures health in terms of one's control over one's personality complex and therefore one's level of awareness or development. Yoga stresses that each assertion of one's 'self' (ego) is a step backward rather than a sign of proper functioning.

There are some other important processes involved with Yoga that are absent in psychology. Yoga believes in karma and reincarnation. Karma is a kind of law of cause and effect in the universe. Very simply it states that you get what you deserve. That is to say, your past actions, both good and bad, result in your present life situation. Now this theory as I have stated it is not so different from what the therapist believes. He too would say that much of an individual's behaviour is determined by previous experience. But what is missing in the West is the notion of reincarnation. With reincarnation one's karma is carried over, or results in another life (or series of lives) under different circumstances. Now the ramifications of this theory are highly significant but too difficult (complicated) for me to go into completely. But briefly, the theory of karma states that man is responsible for both his present and future life situations. If one leads a virtuous life one will be rewarded. If one commits improper behaviour one will be punished. This is one aspect of karma. But there are other related aspects. Yoga says that experience leaves an imprint on one's personality complex. This imprint is called vasana. Vasana is a root-potential — a kind of beginning source. Now when we die and are reborn we are reborn with the same personality complex and spirit. This means that we take our vasanas with us into our next lives. Now psychology talks about instincts and Jung went so far as to outline a collective unconscious. So this theory by Western standards is not so far-fetched when properly understood yet it would definitely be rejected. But the understanding of this aspect of the theory goes a long way towards the understanding of human behaviour. In the West, studies are being done on the XYY factor to show how this leads to criminal behaviour. So the possibility of genetic transfer of behaviour patterns is understood in this sense. So while the psychologist would reject karma and reincarnation on one hand because he cannot observe and measure it, he would accept a genetic theory that states the same thing but with different words.

Now a therapist would not dream of trying to eliminate a patient's instincts. This is not considered possible. The therapist does try to neutralize the impressions that were generated during the childhood experiences of the patient. The yogi, on the other hand, seeks to eliminate all of his vasanas. He seeks to 'burn away' all of his impressions for this and all previous life-times. Now I don't want to get hung up on whether reincarnation is a fact. The significant point here is that the yogi can deal with the very fundamental causes of his behaviour whether he calls them instincts or vasanas or whatever he likes. The therapist is totally incapable of conceiving of such an activity.

The last difference that comes to mind now is Yoga's emphasis upon morality. Yoga, right in the beginning of the process, lays out a moral code that the student must follow if he is even going to begin the process. It is part of the theory behind Yoga that immoral actions disturb the mind. To us in the West this would seem like a very simplistic and childlike idea. We pride ourselves for our new-found moral 'honesty' and rejection of antiquated values. The therapist has helped to foster this trend. Freud rightly pointed to the repressive effects of the Victorian morality of his times. He aptly demonstrated how the super-ego can be the instigating factor behind some neurotic disturbances. But then he and his followers went too far in the other extreme. It was felt that the therapist must adopt a totally non-moral position. It was emphasized that the therapist could not judge his patients if he was to be successful. For this reason some modern writers have said that most analysts would have treated Hitler without trying to stop him in any way. But again I'm straying from the point. I believe that my generation's break from the older generation's morality was in part justified, as hypocrisy was the dominating code of the times. But my generation has not been able to come up with anything better — at least in the sense of attaining any more happiness. I believe this is in part due to the fact that we in the West do not understand the significance of morality. This is also partly due to the fact that those powers — religious leaders — have done badly in their attempts and, as a result, have given morality a 'bad name'. Yoga very easily and graphically shows how morality must be the initial primary concern. But perhaps more important, the yogi himself shows the effects of his moral life.

New Trends in Psychosomatic Medicine

Dr William Kroger

BEFORE BEGINNING my discussion, I should like to define the terms psychosomatic and hypnosis. Psychosomatic refers to the reciprocal and dynamic interaction of emotions and bodily functions in the production of symptoms. Rather than either/or, it is both/and. It does not mean psychologic or psychogenic.

However, more recently the concepts embodied in the term psychosomatic have been expanded to include the environment. Thus, mind-body interrelationships, if one can dichotomize about these, not only react with each other, but continually transact with environmental factors. The behavioural scientist regards the brain as a data processing apparatus which records, stores and retrieves information with amazing rapidity. For instance, it is estimated that the brain contains approximately fifteen billion neurons, each having the capacity to store about 100,000 memories or bits of information. Each cell or neuron has anywhere from one to 1,000 switches or synapses. Now if we multiply fifteen billion by 100,000 by 1,000 this gives us more potential possibilities for combinations of ideas, memories and feelings than there are particles in the universe. This is loosely referred to as the experiential background or subconscious mind. With such a 'channel' capacity and over twenty sensory inputs feeding it, it is no wonder that the brain has been referred to as an 'enchanted loom'.

Contrary to popular opinion, the term hypnosis is not defined as a trance state of sleep or unconsciousness. It is a communication process which enables new learning and understanding to take place more readily than at ordinary levels. This is not at all surprising since whenever a person relaxes, he concentrates better, and thus becomes more receptive to whatever goes to make up the input environment. The hypnotized person develops a hyperacuity to suggestions emanating from within the brain (meditation, prayer, etc.) or from the environment (another person's words, sounds, etc.). It is precisely for this reason that it is used. In other words, whenever the attention span is 'zeroed in' or restricted to specific suggestions, the information 'sinks in'.

The Yoga or Y-State of hypnosis is characterized by a more profound abstraction state. It is produced and maintained by an active effort of the will concentrated on a single idea. Thus, it differs from ordinary hypnosis in that the cerebration is active and controlled and concerned primarily with subjective ideation. In nearly all respects it is similar to the plenary state of hypnotic coma.

During self-reflection, self-absorption, self-contemplation or whatever else one wishes to call auto-hypnosis, the deep meditation leads to insight, self-understanding and tranquility. This is due primarily to increased concentration, turning the attention to the self, and the increasing receptivity to positive and healthy ideas. Where these are repeated again and again, they replace negative, destructive and harmful ideas and thoughts.

In other words, corrective emotional processes are greatly speeded up. Also, viewing the self with greater objectivity allows a better appraisal of one's needs and this leads to greater self-understanding.

There is a growing awareness that all schools of healing for psychosomatic disorders yield approximately the same number of recoveries. Thus, it is obvious that the common denominator of each is faith. Faith is a loaded word and a difficult parameter in man's existence to define. Yet, whenever belief, confidence, motivation and an expectant attitude are catalyzed by the imaginative processes or experiential background, the basis for faith is laid. Now when one belief is compounded upon another belief, this leads to conviction. Hence conviction of cure leads to cure. Nothing could be simpler.

In the genesis of psychosomatic disorders, it is apparent that the psychologic effects are produced by the imagination being stimulated to produce beliefs that are at variance with reality. When these beliefs are reinforced by continually thinking about them, the individual develops the symptom or begins to live the role.

Therefore, the ideal therapy is to reverse this process by either hypnosis or Yoga and get the emotionally disturbed person to imagine — believe — think — and live the idea that he will recover. This might be referred to as the scientific 'power of positive thinking'.

However, I have observed that those who are well conditioned in Yoga do far better than deeply hypnotized persons. It is conceivable that deeper stages of relaxation and concentration more successfully mobilize the adaptive responses. This mechanism appears to tap the 'forgotten assets' or hidden potentials that the sick person ordinarily is unable to call upon to facilitate recovery.

It should be emphasized that recovery arises from an inherent power within the organism. Individuals get themselves sick and they can, in the presence of the proper catalytic agent — the therapist — motivate themselves towards good health. The function of the healer is not to 'play God', but rather to act as a teacher or guide.

It is generally accepted that a high percentage of ailments seen by medical and non-medical healers are of a psychosomatic basis. This indicates that the psychogenic component is largely responsible for the maintenance and dissolution of the symptom. It is generally agreed that all forms of suggestive therapy yield approximately the same number of cures for psychologically based symptoms. Thus, it is obvious that it is not the methodology that is responsible for the healing, but rather the belief, faith, confidence, expectant attitude and motivation that are enhanced as a result of a healthy and strong interpersonal relationship. If this observation is acceptable, then Yoga, hypnosis and other methods which employ autosuggestion will work in direct proportion to the way the patient's beliefs are compounded into conviction.

However, it must be admitted that the meditative state of Yoga leads to a more profound stage of introspection than auto-hypnosis. Thus, this makes possible greater receptivity and objectivity, and consequently newer learnings and richer understanding. The latter has been called everything from nirvana to insight, union with God, and other exalted terms. More simply, it is merely that the increased relaxation and concentration leads to greater self-realization of the individual's problems. By following the four simple tenets of imagining it, believing it, thinking it and living it, a patient can remove a symptom. Interestingly enough, it is these same four principles which induce a psychosomatic symptom. Therefore, all that is necessary is to reverse this process by positive, constructive and healthful reconditioning to replace negative, destructive and harmful conditions.

All suggestive therapies, irrespective of their names, operate on this basis. After all, it is the patient who gets himself sick and it is the patient who gets himself well. The healer merely acts as a catalyst.

Psychosomatic Medicine

Dr Frank Graham

THE TERM PSYCHOSOMATIC in its relationship to disease has come in for some considerable criticism from time to time. The objection has always been that as there is no question that psyche and soma always act as one, why conjure up a term like this; why not just talk of medicine, knowing full well that important psychological factors are present in every disease however physical its effects may be. Whatever the merits of this argument many still hold to the view that the word psychosomatic is useful, particularly in these days when so many are oblivious to the close relationship between mind and body: most of us still think in terms of black and white, either or, the illness is either physical or mental. The term psychosomatic brings into one word these two aspects, thus emphasizing an important unity.

It is hardly possible to study psychosomatic problems without considering the notion of stress and its effects on the individual; of the so-called Unconscious, or that part of the mind that harbours active emotional states albeit out of the range of awareness; of conflict in the mind; of the notion of repression, the mental mechanism by which something unpleasant, distasteful, or unbearable, is rendered unconscious in order to avoid mental pain.

Stress is a mixed blessing. Physical strength could not

develop at all were it not as a response to stress: the weight-lifter by increasing the size of his weights builds bigger and better muscles. Similarly, character develops under stress — the pressure of instinctual needs opposed by the requirements of the family and society — and this implies the need for the development of a strong ego, one that can bear frustration, can tolerate delay in instinctual satisfaction and can bear unpleasant as well as pleasant emotions.

Psychological stress and conflict are present all the time in everyday living. The 'worries' of domestic and business life, the countless decisions of a major and minor nature that are necessary, often run counter to an opposing wish to remain at rest and free from responsibility; the striving towards independence is often in conflict with a strong tendency to remain dependent. What is dangerous to health is not the stress itself so much as its being so prolonged, or too great for the individual's stage of development. What ensures that this state of affairs does not arise is adequate rest, recreation, sleep and relaxation. Regular periods of deliberate conscious relaxation act as a prophylaxis against the development of a chronic state of unrelieved tension which is often the starting point of a psychosomatic disorder.

The ego can be thought of as that part of the mind that registers impressions, makes judgements about the external world and self, seeks out legitimate ways of getting instinctual satisfactions and acts as a dampener on emotionality and instinctual discharge, keeping them within limits. In psychosomatic illnesses there are usually several, sometimes many, simultaneous causes at work, an important one being so-called ego-weakness. A strong ego can experience and hold on to all sorts of unpleasant feelings such as irritation, anger and indignation, sorrow and the unhappy feeling of the loss of a loved-one or something held precious. Sometimes this ego-capacity breaks down and then these distressing emotions tend to spill over, as it were, from the mind into the soma, by way of the autonomic nervous system. Thus we get the bereaved person suffering from a 'heartache' or a 'broken heart'; the chronically frustrated man developing 'ulcer' pains; the business executive who never gets angry with a difficult client having an attack of colitis as soon as the interview is over; the housewife with many irritations in her life who develops an 'irritating' skin condition. In all such instances the ego cannot quite bear in full measure the all-too-upsetting emotional state and finds it much easier to put up with a substitute bodily pain, even though this is also unpleasant. A real danger arises in a possible chronicity of such a state of affairs whereby irreversible changes may occur in the organs concerned.

Thus it is not difficult to understand that early and careful treatment of psychosomatic disorders is important. While this is true, it is well to be aware of possible dangers. For instance, in the treatment of asthma by hypnosis, which is sometimes very helpful, there is a danger of reducing the patient's discomfort so that it no longer acts as a signal of impending oxygen deficiency. Again, patients who have some organic weakness in, for instance, the cardio-vascular system may be precipitated into a heart attack or a stroke by a too vigorous attempt to clear up a psychological problem. However, the above dangers can be exaggerated. Fortunately, with care, the chances of helping a patient are greater than of harming him.

As the factors involved in any single psychosomatic condition are usually multiple, the approach should not be one-sided. Relaxation techniques, meditation, analytical psycho-therapy, group methods, have all an important part to play in strengthening the individual to withstand stress and solve conflicting attitudes. But complete reliance should not be placed on these; except perhaps in the very earliest stages of a disorder, before organic risks or dangers have arisen. Usually attention needs to be paid to environmental factors, infections, allergies, locality; climate and psychological climate both at home and at work.

The question may be asked, just what are the mechanisms involved in bringing about an improvement in a psychosomatic condition by psychological means? This is a fascinating field of study and one that has many theories but not a great deal in the way of hard facts.

However, we are not bereft of some useful ideas on the matter. It seems important to help a patient to be able to rest properly, mentally as well as physically — a problem that affects us more than is generally thought. Again, experience and experiments tend to show that repeated and constant paying of attention to a certain part of the body, or organ, increases the blood flow to that area, and thus improves its function. This points to the usefulness of improving circulation by the study of Yoga and meditation.

The problem of helping a patient solve his conflicts is a more complicated one; and yet it is often an important step towards alleviating his apparently physical symptoms. Both analytical psychotherapy and meditation can be most useful in this way by helping the patient become fully aware of both sides of his conflicts; then, and only then, can one side be disposed of, put out of mind as it were, leaving him free of the tension of a conflict that has persisted owing to too great repression and not enough ventilation.

Freud's later theory concerning Eros (the life instinct) and Thanatos (death instinct), the two principles that govern all living matter may find a valuable application in psychosomatic medicine. The energy of Eros (which binds, unites, integrates) is libido (which is wider than just sex and includes love and other caring emotions); and that of Thanatos (which disintegrates, destroys) is aggression. The two energies always run hand in glove, the former neutralizing the latter. They are thought of as investing every part of the body, every cell, every mental function. Now when some part or organ becomes diseased it can be assumed that libido has been withdrawn from the part leaving it with a surplus of unneutralized destructive aggression. The two questions arise, why was the 'current' of libido withdrawn, and how can it be restored — fundamental research problems.

To what extent psychosomatic symptoms have a 'meaning' has proved a subject of considerable controversy. Can it be said that the ulcer pain really stands for a particular emotional state too difficult to bear; is the patient with the severe diarrhoea or colitis in fantasy trying to expel objects from inside himself felt to be dangerous, or attacking external objects in a fit of hate, wishing to defile or destroy them? It would seem from the analysis of small children and psychotic and prepsychotic adults that these physical symptoms do in fact have specific meanings.

It is another question altogether just what use is made of this knowledge of body-language. To attempt to confront the average adult suffering from a psychosomatic illness with insights of this kind would provoke incredulity, if not outright rejection: a good example of 'wild analysis'. But if the patient in analysis has in time been able to make contact with the deeply buried layers of his mind, these fantasies become more accessible; he is able to see more clearly that they are at times important motivating factors in his life. This is often a crucial step in his developing ego-strength which aids in alleviating the symptoms, and the growth of character.

Psychosomatic factors are always important in disease but they should not be allowed to obscure the equally important somato-psychological complications. The man who suffers a severe heart attack may thereafter be fearful, impotent, feel helpless and lose his former interests. These are somato-psychological effects and should be recognized as such because it may influence the patient's situation. Nevertheless, whichever aspect of the problem seems to be to the fore, psychotherapy is probably the most important one of several approaches to the treatment of a psychosomatic ailment.

Morality and Psychosomatics

Shri Vijayadev Yogendra

RECENT DEVELOPMENTS in the study of psychosomatic medicine have seen a widening of interest by Western scientific thinkers. They are now interested in and willing to learn of Eastern intuitive knowledge in the fields of medicine, psychology and other humanistic sciences. Consequently, they are also interested in the methods of training available in Eastern philosophies that develop the mind. While there are more and more sophisticated research tools being developed, and new areas of investigation opening up to legitimate science, quite often these developments do not contribute to the individual's growth. However, because of these developments, many psychologists, psychiatrists and medical practitioners are looking at the thinking and philosophies of the various cultural, spiritual and religious traditions, to see if they may aid the progress of medical science.

As Dr. Robert Ornstein writes in his book 'The Psychology of Consciousness':

> 'Science as a mode of knowledge involves a limitation of enquiry. The essence of a good experiment is successful exclusion. One factor may be manipulated while a few other processes are measured. If, for example, we want to study the response of cells in the brain to visual stimuli, we would be

> considered mad if we also monitored the blood flow, the temperature of the room, the phase of the moon, the growth of a mushroom outside or any one of the millions of possibilities. But, in psychology of late, the limitations of successful behaviouristic criteria have proven to outweigh the advances. To give one example, psychologists have until recently tended to ignore some evidence from sources as diverse as Yoga and animal experiments, that man is capable of a higher degree of self-mastery of his internal physiology. Further, we have not incorporated the evidence that the linear, verbal and intellectual mode of knowing is not the only mode available to man.'

It is interesting that scientists, psychologists and others are expressing interest in, and trying to assess the results of, the Eastern scientific achievement through empirical tests. However, they constantly run into trouble, for no-one as yet has been able to devise such equipment that will identify and measure this intuitive knowledge definitely. In the case of psychosomatic disorders one factor has constantly emerged most clearly; that is the lack of pathology evidenced in the tests at the onset of the disorder. Even though the patient claims to feel pain, discomfort etc., the investigation does not seem to show any significant variation to register a diseased condition.

Both Eastern and Western authorities accept that psychosomatic disease has a somatic part related to the body, and a psychic part related to the mind. Yet the soul or the spirit is not recognized in modern psychology, psychiatry or psychoanalysis. This creates a stumbling block for Western science. Eastern science recognizes the existence of the spirit or soul, and also the psychic factor in man. This factor has the capacity to override the body-mind complex, and can be trained and treated and thereby overcome conditions of a psychosomatic nature. Furthermore, the Eastern authorities recognize that the causative factors of psychosomatic disorders come from vasanas, or desire-potencies or complexes, which are dormant at a subconscious level and hard to reach through conscious effort. Consequently, they have developed techniques and methods by which they are able to penetrate deep into the subconscious, create the changes essential and necessary to the health of a human being, and so oversome the symptoms of psychosomatic disease.

In the ancient traditions of India, two sciences were recognized by the authorities as being helpful to individuals with conditions of disease — the science of Ayurveda, and the science of Yoga. When an Ayurvedic physician found that a patient's condition was not responding to treatment, he immediately referred him to the yoga authorities, for it is stated in one of the old yogic texts: 'Yoga is the ultimate remedy for those suffering from the problems of existential life'. The subject of Yoga was regarded as a therapeutic science. However, the recommendation to study Yoga was made more for its methods of personal training which enables an individual to discipline and develop himself, integrate his personality and distracted mind, and so attain the highest possible knowledge of the self. In this process his fears, anxieties and tensions were eliminated. Therefore, Yoga and Ayurveda covered the whole field of human requirements and needs. There was no separate branch of psychology in Yoga. There was no need for psychiatry or psychiatric treatment, for the science of Yoga itself covers the area of psychology dealing as it does with the body-mind complex.

Both Yoga and Ayurveda believed in preventive hygiene, and prescribed routines that were comfortable and consistent with the practice of self-discipline. A fixed routine for each day was known as dincharya which aimed to prevent disorder or breakdown. In fact, wherever you find people with a disciplined routine, for example in penal institutions or the army, you will find these people have fewer psychosomatic conditions than those who are not guided by routines or any such discipline. This knowledge was a fact of social science in ancient times. Therefore, in the future, the ideals of social science should recommend to the individual that healthy living must incorporate emotional controls and ethical values, as well as strict routines.

It was also emphasized that when there was a general breakdown in the tone and condition of the human body, strict measures were to be applied in terms of discipline, diet and daily behaviour patterns. In the words of the Founder of The Yoga Institue, Bombay, Shri Yogendra: 'When the homeostatic balance is disturbed either at the physical or mental level, for whatever cause, and when symptoms of disease are evident, immediate action should be taken to restore normalcy. In the case of Ayurveda, this is done through herbal treatment, whereas in the case of Yoga autogenic processes are employed under the guidance of the teacher to re-establish a homeostatic condition.'(2)

The science of Yoga is mainly concerned with the ultimates of diagnosis and cure. It takes a metascientific attitude towards the problems of disease and is mainly interested in its removal from the fundamental point of view, in contrast to the materialistic cash-and-carry programmes of modern medicine. As Dr. Jonas Salk, the eminent medical scientist, has commented: 'Systems like Yoga have much to contribute to our lop-sided development in the field of medicine. The preventive and hygienic aspects of Yoga will have to be studied because Yoga is a science of the healthy man whereas modern medicine is the study of the diseased man. We need more of such science of health to establish true norms for human progress in all areas of life — physical, mental and spiritual.' Thus, the subject of Yoga takes a much broader view of the whole problem of disease and puts forth basic concepts like citta (the total personality complex), karma (action and its consequences), samskara (fundamental tendencies), suddhi (purification) and prana (bioenergy). This holistic approach in Yoga has the capacity to overhaul the whole human machinery and service man at every level of his life and being.

The yoga authority is not satisfied with just understanding the gross body and its management, but is more concerned with the subtle factors involved in the pathogenesis of disease. These subtle factors according to Yoga stem from the psyche, and it is the biological aspects in the psyche that cause the weaknesses of the body. Dr. R.S. Battacharya has rightly said that compelled by the dehadharana samskara the prana indriya (an aspect of the antah karana) transforms the deha visayas of the external objects. The Ayurvedic physicians were right to say that the development of the body is in harmony with the mind, as much as the development of the mind is in harmony with the body. In the words of Shri Yogendra again: 'In the management of disease, Yoga remains non-specific in its approach. At the psychic level, it helps in generating greater sattva, bringing about prajna-consciousness as opposed to prajna-aparadha (error of intellect). With the right approach and a balanced state of mind, it is easier to set up healthy routines and right habits. This is, of course, the yoga way of life which reduces tamasika and rajasika excesses in our personality make-up. Diet (mitahara) also becomes an important factor. 'As is your diet, so is your mind' is an old Ayurvedic adage.' (3)

In this sense, yoga therapy is not just a therapy, but it is by and large a product of personal development. According to Yoga, disease is not the outcome of a single wrong action, but is the outcome of wrong actions compounded in time. Therefore, as a result of going against natural laws by acting in a wrong way, we become victims of the consequences which affect the psyche. Disease comes about as a natural consequence, not because an individual wants or does not want it, but because he has done something contrary to a natural law. The person suffering from disease has to become aware of his wrong actions, and their consequences, before his suffering is relieved. Without this awareness, he will again fall into the same old pattern once he is relieved of the symptom. We see this portrayed in everyday life, where people make mistakes and suffer because of them. The one experience of suffering usually does not make sufficient impact on the individual, who repeats the mistake and continues to suffer. So in trying to understand the factors behind psychosomatic disorders and their evolution, the drive for self-development has to be understood. For it is this drive towards perfection in each individual that begets experiences of suffering, from which an awareness is gradually derived as a means of personal development to fulfil the promise of evolution.

The science of Yoga involves itself with human problems because it believes these problems are problems of life. In their attempts to resolve these problems, the yoga authorities did not look at the superficialities of a disorder, but went to the roots, the seed of the particular disorder. In one of the textbooks of Hatha Yoga it is said that a person suffering from any disorder suffers from three-fold affliction (physical, mental and psychic) and the only remedy is the study of integral Yoga. It is said that the suffering person should be treated consistently and not in part. Therefore, in treating a sick person the yogi will treat him totally, rather than just the part affected. In other words, the yogi who is treating a disease tries to transform his patient by advising, informing and giving guidance that helps the patient to become more integrated and develop a healthier lifestyle. This is why Yoga is defined as a way of life rather than a set of physical jerks, or a pseudo-meditative technique, or method of therapy. Once a person is provided with training he not only eliminates the disorder, but also becomes habituated to a new lifestyle and routine. For as long as he follows the routine meticulously, the discipline of the routine prevents the recurrence of disease.

As mentioned earlier, Yoga sees disease as being three-fold: saririka (biologic or physical), manasika (mental, emotional or intellectual) and adhyatmika (psychic or spiritual). This interrelated syndrome is hardly appreciated by modern science, in the same way that psychic factors are not understood to the extent they should be. There are no qualified physicians who can treat the three-fold aspects of disease, with the exception of the yoga authority. Unfortunately, modern authorities have become so specialized that they know less and less of the whole man.

We see conditions which can be broadly categorized under the headings of headaches, migraines, spinal problems, muscular aches, heart conditions, blood pressure, tension, hypertension, digestive and various other disorders. All these have a basis that can be linked to a condition of the mind, in particular, the emotional aspect. Therefore, it is not easy to define what exactly goes under the category of psychosomatic disease, and what does not. However, many people are inclined to believe that eighty per cent of disease conditions belong to the psychosomatic group. If this is the case, then we have to understand the approaches made by both Eastern and Western authorities in curing these disorders.

Naturally every individual is interested in what is a cure. In many cases psychosomatic ailments fool many people, who give up hope and suffer for a lifetime. In Yoga, cure is made possible through the gradual assimilation of fundamental rather than transient values, and cleansing the body of toxic materials in the vital organs, restoring the homeostatic balance and creating poise (samatva). One singularly important factor in the treatment of disease in Yoga is finding the cause-potentials which affect the various planes of life. Today, psychiatrists are naturally interested in finding the causes. However, when investigating the cause-potentials of consciousness one has to go beyond the conscious to be able to reach and read the subconscious, and relate it to what the individual exhibits as an outward manifestation of disease. Here one must recognize the fact that this secret chamber of men and women is crammed with worldly thoughts and ideas, and with desires. The subconscious plane is a vast field possessing huge amounts of power and possibilities. It is also a hidden storehouse of energy. As a matter of fact all powers that are manifested in the physical, mental and spiritual planes are different phases of the same unmanifested energy lying latent in the subconscious of man. This search for cause-potential is one of the most important aspects of yoga technology, if at all such a term should be used in understanding Yoga.

Apart from this search for cause-potential, the yoga authorities took measures on the physical plane. Consequently, yoga therapeutic techniques are a by-product of its hygienic and preventive education for all aspects of the human being — physical, mental, emotional, moral and spiritual. In this way control of the mind is made possible, and a person is able to carry through a positively oriented programme that helps him live a healthy and disease-free life.

Now when we look at the treatment of psychosomatic disorders in Eastern and Western approaches we come across one common denominator. It can be seen that both Eastern and Western authorities agree that a person in a state of relaxation is able to temporarily relieve his symptoms, or even overcome his condition of disease. I have observed this many times when people come to me with bad attacks of asthma. I sit them in my office, and talk about matters which are pleasing to them, or take away their attention from themselves by introducing a humorous topic, or something to involve their interest. Slowly as they focus their attention on my conversation or approach they relax, and, as if in a lulled condition of mind, broaden their area of attention. Their concentration is diverted from their condition, releasing them from their self-centredness, and thus they find themselves less distressed in breathing. This process has been noticed by members of the healing professions in the East and West. Therefore, relaxation has been the key factor in the treatment of psychosomatic conditions.

However, either one is able to relax temporarily for a few minutes, or a few hours, or one can find a way of relaxing permanently. This permanency can only be achieved through a mental attitude which is relaxed and therefore confident. This attitude immediately changes the individual's metabolism. Studies throughout the world are now being made with cases of high blood pressure, coronary disease and asthma, where individuals are induced into a deep state of relaxation, which in turn brings about relief. Some people have even claimed that they have been able to effectively cure cancer by bringing about such a state of deep relaxation. Some use methods of hypnosis, others have found great advantage in using the methods of Schultz called autogenic training (which are no more and no less than the simple relaxation techniques of Yoga).

But relaxation cannot be treated as a separate aspect which is what Western psychologists, psychiatrists and medical practitioners are doing. They link techniques of relaxation to the superficialities of the mind at a conscious level. Yet some are trying to penetrate beyond the conscious to understand and relax the subconscious. Most think relaxation is something which need not be taught in conjunction with moral and ethical principles although they influence a person's whole being by bringing about a relaxed state of mind. A person can be asked to lie down and relax, and he will relax. But if he has not the necessary moral fibre his relaxation will be only skin-deep and not a deep relaxation which is the only way a person can overcome a psychosomatic illness.

According to Yoga, relaxation cannot be taught to a person who has emotional tension, is under stress, either consciously or subconsciously, or is fearful, anxious, apprehensive or doubtful. Inevitably such a person cannot attain the desired state of relaxation, although he may enjoy piece-meal relaxation. In order to overcome this emotional condition of tension one has to find where the emotionalism comes from; whether it comes from fear, anxiety or any other factor which is related to mundane involvement in life, the senses or the egoistic factor of an individual.

However, we believe that if a person is trained to follow some fundamental values that are natural, universal and permanent, he becomes more confident in himself, knowing fully that he is following only those values which will not be overtaken by time or be unacceptable to society. These permanent values or natural laws are derivations from the fundamental primordial laws of Nature, which have been given to us by the Prophets and Saviours as moral and ethical codes. These people have come and gone, have propounded the application of morality and shown by their example what can be achieved through the state of concentration and relaxation. We, who are more scientifically minded, have accepted them but never allowed ourselves to believe moral values have any influence on an individual's state of health or his capacity for relaxation. Therefore, we have by-passed them, ignored them, and ridiculed them and their moral teachings.

From my observation and experience the more a person is rooted in his sense of morality, the more he is free from anxiety and tension, the greater is the state of relaxation. In achieving this state a person progresses, as he conquers his fears, anxieties, insecurities and lack of confidence which are the roots of any and every psychosomatic disorder.

In yoga technology the yoga authorities define five states or levels of mental activitiy (citta bhumi). The first state is known as ksipta in which the mind is under the domination of the rajas and tamas gunas, unstable gunas which result in the mind being attracted to the objects of the senses and conditions of excitability. The second state is mudha in which there is an excess of excitability and a tendency towards sensualism, lethargy and dormancy. The third phase of the mind is known as viksipta where the mind is distracted and irritable etc. This state has hardly any beneficial influences. In this state, however, there is temporary concentration of citta but the mind is still very easily distracted. The fourth state is ekagrata or concentration in which the mind is trained and disciplined, where the impurities of the mind are eliminated and there is a manifestation of more positive elements. In this state the possibility of prolonged concentration on one object is realized. Lastly they talk of the state of niruddha in which there is a cessation of mental modifications and total concentration is available to the person who is attempting to follow the yoga way of life. It is in this state that a person exhibits the state of complete relaxation.

Another aspect of yoga technology is its understanding of the phenomenon of human energy or bioenergy (prana). It can be found that the improvement of the energy ratio or balance has a very direct effect on psychosomatic conditions. The prana or bioenergy relates to the primal cosmic energy outside the electro-magnetic spectrum and other forces known to Western science. The acupuncturists call it chi, the Greeks called it ether, Christianity refers to it as the 'breath of life' as described in Genesis Chapter II, the Russian psychic research scientists have dubbed it 'bioplasma', and dozens more terms could be found for the same basic energy that permeates all living organisms. It is the source of all vital activity including thought, feeling, perception, movement, etc. Therefore, it would be difficult not to accept this 'living force', which acts intelligently and purposefully, and controls the activities of every molecule of living matter. We must accept that it carries life principles from one place to another, overhauling and purifying neurons and maintaining the subtle life-giving areas of the body in the same way the blood plasma maintains the gross body. A greater amount of research is necessary to establish the essence of this energy and how it is extracted by the nervous system from the tissues. In human beings this essence especially relates to the vitality of the individual.

We can say that the human mind, which is not the citta, is nothing but the continual associated acclimatization to environments. The more perfect the acclimatization, the more perfect is the manifestation of life. The law of acclimatization is not mechanical or chemical but what we call the manifestation of life force or prana. Everything seems to be governed by this law and it is the violation of this law which brings disorder to the body and the psyche. It also brings ill-health or disease. Therefore the fulfilment of this tendency and the establishment of perfect harmony with the environment and obeying of the natural law are implicit in the meaning of acclimatization.

We can therefore assume that health means life under natural conditions where the law of cellular intelligence and other laws that govern the environment are not violated. So if the acclimatization is imperfect the result is ill-health or disease. Disease is not a real entity that attacks us from time to time but is simply imperfection in the manifestation of life-force or prana. It is this inability of the life sustaining force to acclimatize itself to its given environment. We all know that we need a certain amount of energy to acclimatize ourselves to the surrounding conditions whether internal or external; but when we are short of the requirement of the energy-complex as the energy has been drained either by waste or dissipation or by violation of hygienic laws, we grow weak and are unable to resist the external influences and succumb to various ailments. For example, if the outside temperature drops to freezing and we fail to acclimatize to that change we are surely going to get cold etc. If we are not able to acclimatize to an intake of too rich a diet then indigestion must overtake us. But instead if we have enough energy or vitality in us we can overcome the factors which demand change and our resources are able to stimulate such psycho-chemical activity to enable us to remain healthy. So one can say what we call a naturally healthy person is no more or less than the effect of bioenergy and its stable influence on the body-mind complex.

It is commonly found that people who have emotional problems are normally devitalized, lacking in energy, have an imbalanced distribution of energy and consequently function inharmoniously. Sometimes they have an excess of uncontrolled energy, for example, anger, which is self-destructive and self-defeating. Under the natural law the flow of energy in the individual is towards the external world, which means he loses his energy through the senses to the outside world. In the study of Yoga the energy is turned within to the inner self and is reunited with the subtle spiritual energies. This reinforcement of the life-force into the whole system of the human body creates the spiritual growth, deep relaxation and a totality of development that prevents psychosomatic illness.

This total energy complex in an individual could be termed 'universal energy' as it also pervades the entire universe. In the human body it is more specific, having five-fold functions or currents. The first is prana which is mainly an upholder as its job is to harmonize the whole functioning of the body. Then there is apana or the force that eliminates toxicity from the body. Then vyana where circulation is the main function. Samana is the current which is associated with assimilation in the body and udana is associated with metabolism both catabolic and anabolic. The collective name for the currents is prana and the proper functioning of prana maintains good health, vitality and life itself. The practice of the yoga pranayama techniques becomes very important because they control the force and elements that create a healthy body.

Equivalents to prana or bioenergy can be found in electricity, in heat, light, gravitation and magnetism. All these phenomena are expressions of energy. In the human body the energy flows through nerves and hence it is called nervous energy, in the muscles it becomes muscular energy and in the sexual organs it becomes sexual energy. In its finer forms it becomes mental power, will power, thought power, the power of imagination, understanding, etc. In a body with good health there is balance of prana in the nerves (nadis). When this balance is disturbed through wrong ways of living or thinking, or there is an accumulation of toxic material or obstruction of the nerves, the flow of prana is disrupted causing diseases and loss of vitality and personality control.

This bioenergy is affected by every shade of passion, emotion, by our intake of food and drink, by the environment and our mode of life. In fact, it is affected by all the thousands of influences, from the most powerful to the slightest, that act to shape life from birth to death. Thus the need for a balanced, moral way of living is based on a biological imperative.

In Yoga there is no uniformity of technique for diagnosing disease or its treatment. The yogi does not use any modern instruments in diagnosis, but relies heavily on his personal experience and intuition. The recent attempts to bring instruments and to record their readings thereby diagnosing the disease prevents the medical practitioner — who is not recognized by the yogi — from seeing that it is a subtle working of the whole body which causes disease. Even though the yoga authority does not use the modern scientific instrumentation for his diagnosis, he is capable of diagnosing correctly on the basis of his intuition and experience of each individual. He is able to sense in each individual the total content of his energy complex.

One has to accept the fact that the modern scientific-minded medical practitioner looks for a type of therapy that can be prescribed uniformly. This is not accepted in

Yoga because yoga therapy operates as a process of education where the relationship between the teacher and student is a very personal thing. What passes between them, and its measured impact, cannot be found in a textbook nor can it be generalized for mass use. To the yogi, each individual is separate and is treated by him on the merits and demerits of his case by applying to the particular case the fundamental laws he has learnt. This is not acceptable to the Western scientist, and therefore he wants to use his instruments to assess and evaluate the work of a yogi. This is impossible to do, and even the work that is done is carried out with the usual scepticism. The yoga authority should be unconcerned with this attitude — that everything has to be proven. The main thing is that a solution is found and the condition alleviated or cured. What is more important is that more people should undertake a training in self-development and find a basis in values. In the long run this would create benevolent people who would help their fellow human beings out of an immense interest in caring for and loving them. This is something that will be accepted in generations to come. However, because we are technologically and scientifically oriented, it is hard just yet to accept this basis for the treatment of psychosomatic disorders.

In my personal study I have observed that most diseases are caused because of a lack of love and compassion (maitreya and karuna), of an incapacity to love or give or serve, due to ignorance (agyana) or an overemphasis on greed and the satisfaction of desires that a person generates in a lifetime. The desires trigger off an imbalanced condition which contributes to the development of guilts, feelings of anxiety, fear and resentment among others. Every event in our life is closely linked to the energy index. Happiness, fear, anxiety, anger, etc, cause changes in our heart beat, in our gastro-intestinal tract and in the secretions of the various glands. All this affects the human condition so that one part of the body is deprived at the cost of another to sustain an energy index.

What happens in the human body as an individual progresses in age, is that the body is subjected to constant wear and tear due to the emotions. Characteristically, weakness and susceptibility develop in the nerves and cells. This results in a lack of absorption, maintenance, repair and growth in the various parts of the body's physiology. All these things culminate in a disease, or cause a symptom of disease. It is for this reason that an individual is advised to practise self-restraint to protect himself from fluidity of mind or over-anxiety, which in turn protects himself from precipitating degeneration and disease.

It is a fact that in the practice of psychosomatic medicine, the wisdom of the healer cures the disease, and not the medicine. Until Western medical practitioners, psychologists, psychiatrists and counsellors accept this basic fact, any attempt in bringing about a permanent change in a person's psychosomatic illness will not be successful. Therefore in order to be a good therapist one must be spiritually developed, gathering within oneself complete knowledge, but above all, developing a full capacity to relax and concentrate, give, care and be available at any time to those in need of attention and passing the same on to others.

1. Ornstein, Dr. R. 'The Psychology of Consciousness', W.H. Freeman & Co., San Francisco (1972) p. 6.
2. Yogendra, Shri 'Yoga and Therapy', The Yoga Institute, Bombay (1977) p. 10.
3. ibid p. 10.

Biographical Notes

Dempster, Dr Alec

Dr Dempster is Trainee Liason Officer with the Family Medical Programme of the Royal Australian College of General Practitioners as well as a General Practitioner.

Dugal, Dr Satya Pal

Dr Duggal holds degrees in Sanskrit (M.A.), Chemistry (M.Sc.) and Education (M.Ed.). He also is a qualified teacher of Yoga (C.T.Y.Ed.) from The Yoga Institute, Bombay. Dr Duggal is Professor of Teaching at the S. L. Training College in India and is also the author of numerous books including 'Psychology in Education' and 'Manual of Education Guidance and Counselling'.

Dugan, Jan

Graduated from the University of Melbourne in 1966 with the degree of Bachelor of Arts and, later, obtained a Dip. Psych. She has worked as a Clinical Psychologist for ten years and is now a Student Counsellor at Swinburne Institute of Technology, Melbourne.

Dugan, Patrick

A student of Yoga for over ten years, Mr Dugan teaches

part-time at the Yoga Education Centre. He also holds a M.Sc. degree and Dip.Ed. He has taught biology at Prahran High School and is now the Principal of The Helen Vale Foundation School of Total Education.

Graham, Dr Frank

Dr Graham is a Fellow of the Royal College of Psychiatrists. He has been practising for over thirty years both in Australia and overseas. He is currently Medical Psychoanalyst at the Prince Henry's Hospital, Melbourne.

French, Dr Ronald

Educated at Wesley College and Melbourne University. Graduated with Bachelor of Dental Science in 1946. Dr French entered general dental practice in 1947. He graduated as Doctor of Dental Surgery, University of Toronto, 1963. Fellow of the Royal Australian College of Dental Surgeons, 1965.

Gudkovs, Janet

Graduated from the University of Melbourne in 1973 with an honours degree in Psychology. Her honours thesis dealt with personality development. She now works as a counsellor for The Helen Vale Foundation and teaches part-time at the Yoga Education Centre, Melbourne.

Ingbritsen, Kenneth

Mr Ingbritsen holds a degree in Town Planning from the University of Melbourne. He was formerly the President of Social Involvement at the University of Melbourne and the National Director of A.U.S. Social Action. He is now the Secretary of The Helen Vale Foundation, of which he is also a Director.

Kenghe, Dr C.T.

Dr Kenghe is Reader in Sanskrit at Aligarh University, India. He is a renowned scholar and has written many works on Yoga and Yoga Psychology.

Kroger, Dr William

Formerly Associate Professor of Obstetrics and Gynaecology, Chicago Medical School, and Past President of the Academy of Psychosomatic Medicine.

Maddison, Professor David

Born in 1927. After completing his schooling at Sydney Grammer School he attended the University of Sydney, where he graduated in 1948, (M.B. B.S. Hons.). In 1955 he became a member of the Royal Australasian College of Physicians and was elected a Fellow in 1963. In 1964 he was made a foundation Fellow of the Royal Australian and New Zealand College of Psychiatrists. He is now Dean of the Faculty of Medicine at the University of Newcastle.

Mander, Dr David

A student of Yoga for over thirteen years, Dr David Mander is the Senior Men's Teacher at the Yoga Education Centre, Melbourne. He holds a Ph.D. in Mathematics from Monash University.

Otsuka, Dr Yasuo

Dr Otsuka is one of Japan's leading exponents of traditional Chinese medicine. He is the Director of the Ktiasato Medical Research Institute, Tokyo, and Director of the Japanese Society of Oriental Medicine. He has written numerous papers and articles dealing with the methods and principles of traditional Chinese medicine.

Pawsey, Dr John

A General Practitioner for nearly 28 years, Dr Pawsey has written numerous articles on medical practice. He is aslo on the School Council for the Helen Vale Foundation School of Total Education and the Advisory Council of the Helen Vale Foundation Psychosomatic and Counselling Centre.

Sherman, Dr Robert

Dr Sherman holds a Ph.D. in Psychology and is a practising psychologist. He has studied at The Yoga Institute, Bombay, and is qualified to teach Yoga.

Sharma, Pandit Shiv

Born in 1906. Pandit Shiv Sharma studied for many years under his father, Ram Prasad Sharma, the famous Indian Ayurvedic physician and surgeon. He became the youngest person ever to be appointed Professor of Ayurveda at the Lahore College of Ayurveda. He is the Chairman of the Task Force on Indian Medicine for the Fifth Year Plan and also President of the Central Council of Indian Medicine.

Walters, Dr John

Dr Walters (M.B. B.S.) completed his medical studies at the University of Melbourne in 1972 and has since served as a General Practitioner. He is the Honorary Director of the Helen Vale Foundation's Department of Counselling and Psychosomatic Medicine, and also teaches part-time at the Yoga Education Centre, Melbourne.

Yogendra, Dr Jayadev

Dr Jayadev holds both B.A. (Hons) and M.A. degrees. He gained a Ph.D. for a prize-winning thesis on Samkhya and Yoga. He is currently the Principal of the Teacher Training Academy at The Yoga Institute and is the editor of 'The Journal of The Yoga Institute'.

Yogendra, Shri Vijayadev

Shri Vijayadev was the Registrar and Senior Lecturer at The Yoga Institute, Bombay, before he settled in Australia in 1964. He is the Director of the Yoga Education Centre, Melbourne, and is President of the Yoga Teachers Federation of Australia. Shri Vijayadev inspired the formation and growth of The Helen Vale Foundation and is its Chairman. He is also a member of the Board of Governors of the International Board of Yoga. He is the editor of the 'Journal of the Helen Vale Foundation' and 'Yoga Quarterly', now in its twelfth year of publication.

Yogendra, Shri

Born in 1897. In 1916 he was introduced to Yoga by the famous Yogin Paramahamsa Madhavadasaji. He lived for over two years at the latter's hermitage. Subsequently he founded The Yoga Institute in 1918 and then spent three years in Europe and the U.S.A. spreading the message of scientific Yoga. He has published over thirty works some of which were selected as the best books of the twentieth century to be read after 6,000 years in the Crypt of Civilization. In 1971 he was appointed the Honorary President of the International Board of Yoga. He is a registered medical practitioner and President of The Yoga

Institute. He has been an editor of 'The Journal of The Yoga Institute' since it was first published over thirty years ago.

Glossary

Allopathy: Conventional western medical system.

Angina: Paroxysmal chest pain caused by inadequate blood and oxygen supply to the heart.

Asana: Yoga physical education (physiological practices).

Ayurveda: An indigenous system of medical science developed in India. Literally the 'science of life'.

Blood Pressure [B.P.]: The pressure of the blood against the walls of the arteries. It is expressed as maximum pressure (systolic) over minimum pressure (diastolic).

Citta: The perceptual mechanism.

Colitis: Inflammation of the large intestine or colon.

EEG [Electroencephalogram]: A method of recording the electrical activity of the brain.

Endocrine Glands: Ductless organs that secrete hormonal substances internally into the bloodstream.

Gunas: Constituents of primal matter.

Hatha Yoga: Physiological Yoga.

Homeostasis: The tendency of normal body states to stabilize.

Hypertension: High blood pressure.

Hypotensive Therapy: Treatment to lower blood pressure.

Kapha: Alkaline secretions.

Karma: The cycle of action and reaction.

Manas: Mind consciousness.

Neuron: The nerve cell or structural unit of the nervous system.

Patanjali: Author of the Yoga Sutras.

Pitta: Bile or acid secretions.

Pranayama: Regulation, conservation and control of the bio-energy.

Pratyahara: Abstraction.

Psoriasis: A chronic inflammatory skin disease.

Rajas: One of the constituents of primal matter.

Samskara: Impression in the mind stuff.

Sattva: One of the constituents of primal matter.

Tamas: One of the constituents of primal matter.

Thyrotoxicosis: Disease resulting from overactivity of the thyroid gland.

Unani: A system of medical science practised in Arabic countries.

Vasana: Desire potencies.

Vata: Heat.

Vital Capacity: The volume of air that can be expelled from the lungs by the most forcible expiration after the deepest inspiration.

Yoga Sutras: A treatise on the metaphysics of Yoga.

Index

abstraction, 29
acupuncture, 119
aggression, 139
alcohol, 24
alienation, 17
allopathy, 101
anger, 23, 116
angina, 69-70
anxiety, 11-19, 21, 46, 61, 69, 80, 82, 168
apthous ulcers, 63
art, 101
asana, 29, 47, 48
asthma, 46, 71-72, 154, 166
atman, 115
attitudes, 22, 45, 47, 53, 55, 70
ayurveda, 83, 101, 102, 106-113, 160, 162

back pain, 51
bioenergy, 29, 133, 162, 169-174
biofeedback, 24
blood pressure, 164, 166
body-mind complex, 52, 81, 159
breathing, techniques of, 29, 47, 69, 71
bruxism, 60, 64, 65
buddhi, 125

cancer, 166
character, 60, 78, 84, 132, 157
chinese medicine, 114-120
choice, 11-14
citta, 124, 162
colitis, 46, 154, 156
collective unconscious, 128
community, 16
concentration, 24, 29, 32, 54-55, 134, 148, 150, 168
conditioning, 22, 48-49
conjunctivitis, 72
consciousness, 138, 142, 143
contemplation, 135
contentment, 53
counselling, 92-93

dental problems, 59-65
detribalized, 11, 17
depression, 19, 26, 63, 80
dharana, 29
diarrhoea, 23, 156
diary, 38, 56-57
diet, effect of, 106, 162
disease, definition of, 31, 163
discipline, 38, 57
disposition, 45
dosha, 107-108
drugs, 50, 65

ectomorth, 108
education, emotional, 26-30
education, psycho-physical, 28
ego, 140, 142, 143, 153-154
emotional reactions, 22, 23, 27, 28, 48, 53, 59, 61
emotional disturbance, 44,

46, 72
emotional education, 26-30
emotional reactions, 22, 23, 27, 28, 48, 53, 59, 61
emotions, 27, 110, 115, 125, 173-174
endomorph, 108
environment, 84
Eros, 155-156
existential, 19

faith, 149
fear, 45-46, 52
food, 39-40
Freud, 126-127, 128, 155

gastrointestinal complaints, 63
gestalt, 140
God, 131
guilt, 52, 80

hayfever, 71
headaches, 51
health, 27, 37, 44, 140
heart attack, 157
heart disease, 164, 166
hippocrates, 107
homeostasis, 102, 161
humanity, in medicine, 82-90
humour, 107
hypertension, 69
hypnosis, 29, 148-150

id, 140
immorality, 111
indigestion, 51
insomnia, 63, 65, 68

Jung, 144

kapha, 107-108
karma, 145, 162
ki, 114-119

libido, 156
lifestyle, 52
listening, 49, 56
love, 87-89; 174
  lack of, 173

manas, 124
medical practitioners, 82-90
medicine, chinese, 114-120
medicine, traditional, 118
meditation, 132, 155
mental disease, 111, 140
mesomorph, 108
migrains, 164
mind, 48, 51, 52, 66-68, 112, 122, 124-125, 133, 143, 147, 152, 164, 168,
  training of, 54, 56
moral, principles, 24, 29, 50,
  way of life, 29, 67
morality, 13, 145-146,
  and psychosomatics, 158-174
motives, 38
mouth, the, 60
mouth ulcers, 63

negative attitudes, 68, 78
negative thinking, 52
neuralgia, 63
neurotic, 18
nispanda bhava, 49

pain, 60-63
Patanjali, 123-127, 131, 132, 133
patience, 53
perserverance, 53
personal unconscious, 130
personality, 21
  deterioration of, 23
  development of, 60, 78
physical education, 28
pitta, 107-108
pneuma, 115
prana, 115, 133, 162,

169-174
pranayama, 29, 47, 48
pratyahara, 29
psoriasis, 46
psyche, 29, 109, 110, 111, 114, 115, 162
psychic, 159
psychic diseases, 103, 117
psychic powers, 130
psychology and yoga, 121-136, 137-146
psychosomatic disorders, 14, 83, 151,
basis of, 22, 23, 45, 46
cure of, 47, 69
definition of, 31, 44, 51 106-107, 147, 152, 159
dental, 59-65
moral aspects, 158-174
prevention of, 54, 92
and yoga, 102-105
psycho-physical, 28
psychotropic drugs, 18

rajas, 123, 125
reality, nature of, 137, 141, 143
reincarnation, 145
relaxation, 24, 29, 42, 56, 67, 150, 153, 166-168
routines, 37-43, 161, 164

samskara, 162
samana, 171
sattva, 123
science, 101
self, concept of, 33, 129, 131, 171
self-acceptance, 33, 53
self-awareness, 23, 90
self-control, 42
self-discipline, 50, 54
self-esteem, 15-16, 17, 60
self-observation, 47
self-respect, 81
self-undertsanding, 48
sex, 11, 141, 142
Sigmund Freud, 126
skin pallor, 23
soma, 29, 31, 152
somatic, 115
sore throat, 151
soul, 122-123
spiritual development, 40, 171
spirituality, 94
stress, 24, 63, 64, 82, 107, 152, 153
subconscious, 21, 22, 23, 46, 147, 165, 167
sublimation, 141-142
suddhi, 162
suffering, 78, 81
superego, 126
superego, 126, 140, 145
sweating, 23

tamas, 123, 125
teeth, 60
temporomandibular-joint pain, 63
tension, 20-25, 28, 48, 49, 54, 63, 66, 80, 82, 127, 130, 168
tension, teeth, 60-61, 64, 65
Thanatos, 155-156
theotherapy, 102
thyrotoxicosis, 72
traditional medicine, 118
tridosha, concept of, 107-109

ulcers, 154, 156
ulcers, mouth, 63
unani, 101
unconscious, 28, 33, 126, 127, 128, 152

weakness, 23

valium, 65
vasana, 144, 160

vayu, 107-108

yoga, 24, 29, 42, 70, 71, 72-73, 155
- and hypnosis, 148
- and psychology, 121-136, 137-146
- and psychosomatics, 102
- teacher of, 47
- techniques of, 44-50
- therapy of, 101-105, 158-174

Yogendra Nispanda Bhava, 49
yogi, 112